the
Paleo
Gut Healing
Cookbook

75 Nourishing Paleo + AIP-Friendly
Recipes with 10 Must-Have Practices
to Strengthen Digestion and
a 14-Day Gut Refresh Meal Plan

ALISON MARRAS

FAIR WINDS

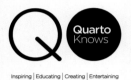

Inspiring | Educating | Creating | Entertaining

Brimming with creative inspiration, how-to projects, and useful information to enrich your everyday life, Quarto Knows is a favorite destination for those pursuing their interests and passions. Visit our site and dig deeper with our books into your area of interest: Quarto Creates, Quarto Cooks, Quarto Homes, Quarto Lives, Quarto Drives, Quarto Explores, Quarto Gifts, or Quarto Kids.

© 2021 Quarto Publishing Group USA Inc.
Text © 2021 Alison Marras

First Published in 2021 by Fair Winds Press,
an imprint of The Quarto Group,
100 Cummings Center, Suite 265-D,
Beverly, MA 01915, USA.
T (978) 282-9590 F (978) 283-2742 QuartoKnows.com

Fair Winds Press titles are also available at discount for retail, wholesale, promotional, and bulk purchase. For details, contact the Special Sales Manager by email at specialsales@quarto.com or by mail at The Quarto Group, Attn: Special Sales Manager, 100 Cummings Center, Suite 265-D, Beverly, MA 01915, USA.

25 24 23 22 21   1 2 3 4 5

ISBN: 978-0-7603-7133-6

Digital edition published in 2021
eISBN: 978-0-7603-7134-3

Library of Congress Cataloging-in-Publication Data available.

Design: Samantha J. Bednarek,
samanthabednarek.com
Cover Image: Alison Marras
Page Layout: Samantha J. Bednarek,
samanthabednarek.com
Photography: Alison Marras

Printed in China

The information in this book is for educational purposes only. It is not intended to replace the advice of a physician or medical practitioner. Please see your healthcare provider before beginning any new health program.

Dedication

For my Abuelo, who ignited my passion for food as medicine and whose support I still carry in my heart today. To my husband, Demetrios, and daughter, Irene Alexandra, who nourish me beyond what food ever could, every single day. And to the supportive readers of FoodbyMars.com.

FOREWORD

Every human cell is impacted by the activities of our gut microbes. A healthy gut microbial community is essential for our health. In fact, about 90 percent of all diseases (including autoimmune disease) can be traced back to the health of the gut and our gut microbiomes. Additional gut-health linked conditions are as wide-ranging as cancer, obesity, diabetes, cardiovascular disease, anxiety, depression, neurodegenerative diseases, autism, ulcers, liver disease, gout, PCOS, osteoporosis, systemic infections, allergies, asthma, and the list continues.

Nourishing the root of our health, *our gut health,* is vital to the prevention and support of such conditions. Our gut microbes perform many different essential functions that help us to stay healthy. These include digestion, vitamin production, detoxification, control of gut barrier integrity, regulation of cholesterol metabolism, providing resistance to pathogens, immune regulation, neurotransmitter regulation, regulation of gene expression, and more! In fact, our gut microbiome can be considered a virtual organ, so it's easy to see that supporting gut health is essential for our overall health.

Experts are increasingly recognizing that certain dietary factors are key contributors to many chronic illnesses—including autoimmune disease and lifestyle-related diseases such as type 2 diabetes, cardiovascular disease, and obesity—mediated, at least in part, through the interaction between the foods we eat and the health of our guts. The use of "food as medicine" is something I've been pioneering for almost a decade, and much of this work has been centered around the Paleo and AIP (Autoimmune Protocol) diets.

Paleo is a nutrient-focused whole-foods diet, with the goal to maximize foods that heal and minimize foods that harm. It improves health by providing balanced and complete nutrition while avoiding most processed and refined foods and empty calories. Contrary to the modern USDA dietary guidelines that have led the public astray for decades, Paleo aims to restore our bodies to nature. And, it's not a quick fix or magic pill diet that so many of us have been fed over the years . . . it's not a fad that dissolves under scientific scrutiny; rather, every Paleo principle is solidly rooted in the latest research and data.

The Autoimmune Protocol is a therapeutic version of the Paleo template designed to help regulate the immune system, mitigating autoimmune and other chronic diseases using key elimination, reintroduction, and maintenance phases. There have been several clinical trials conducted with the use of AIP for conditions such as inflammatory bowel disease (2017) and Hashimoto's Thyroiditis (2019) showing a significant reduction in symptoms. This reinforces that autoimmune disease activity is directly linked to our food choices and how we decide to live our lives. And, while the AIP is not a substitute for medical intervention, this also highlights how those of us with autoimmune disease can regain our health by changing what we eat and making more informed choices about sleep, activity, and stress . . . and that's some pretty darned good news!

Here's more good news: using the Paleo and Autoimmune Protocol principles to advance your healing journey doesn't have to be stressful, overwhelming, or bland. You can harness these effective tools while having fun in the kitchen and finding balance in your life with the right knowledge and support. And that's where *The Paleo Gut Healing Cookbook* comes in!

Alison brings her personal and professional experience, combined with her love of food into this approachable cookbook, jam-packed with *delicious* recipes! She's making a gut-healthy lifestyle more practical, breaking down the foundations for you so it's attainable and joyful. While the diet and recipe aspect is a huge component of this cookbook, so are the leading chapters to help set you up for success. Alison also helps you put everything you learn here into practice with the included two-week meal plan and additional resources.

With this cookbook, Alison will inspire you to take control of your health with delicious, eclectic flavors, recreating your (and her) favorites like Puerto Rican Pastelón, Greek Moussaka, Chicken Pad Thai, and Coconut Custard Pie just to name a few. She'll sneak gut-healing foods like broths, ferments, and prebiotic-rich vegetables into meals you wouldn't imagine using them in like Hot Cocoa Bone Broth and introduce you to healing herbs, especially using the Drinks and Tonics chapter while teaching you "why" along the way! Expect to feel well-fed and empowered using this beautiful and indispensable resource on your gut health journey with Paleo.

—Dr. Sarah Ballantyne, Ph.D., *New York Times* best-selling author of *The Paleo Approach*

CONTENTS

INTRODUCTION   8

CHAPTER 1
Gut Healing with Paleo   11

CHAPTER 2
10 Everyday Practices
for Optimal Digestion   23
How to Use This Book   49

CHAPTER 3
Soups & Stews   55

CHAPTER 4
Entrées   79

CHAPTER 5
Veggies & Sides   117

CHAPTER 6
Salads   139

CHAPTER 7
Desserts   151

CHAPTER 8
Drinks & Tonics   165

CHAPTER 9
Staples & Condiments   181

CHAPTER 10
2-Week Gut Refresh Meal Plan   196

ABOUT THE AUTHOR   200
ACKNOWLEDGMENTS   200
RESOURCES & REFERENCES   201
INDEX   204

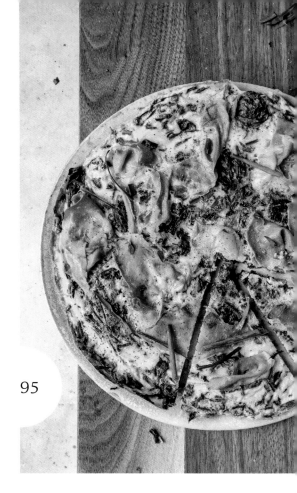

95

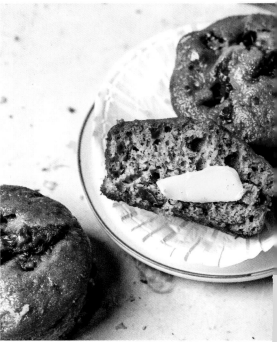

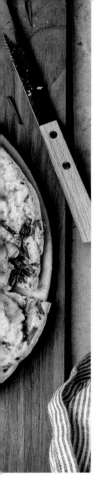

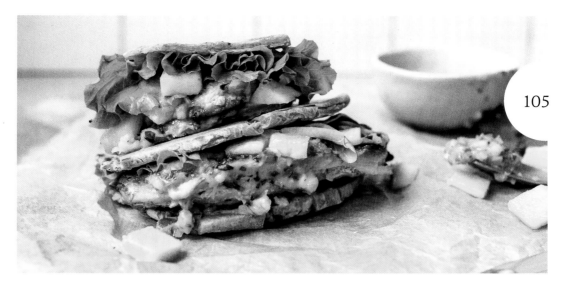

105

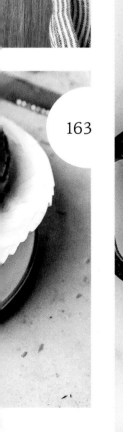

163

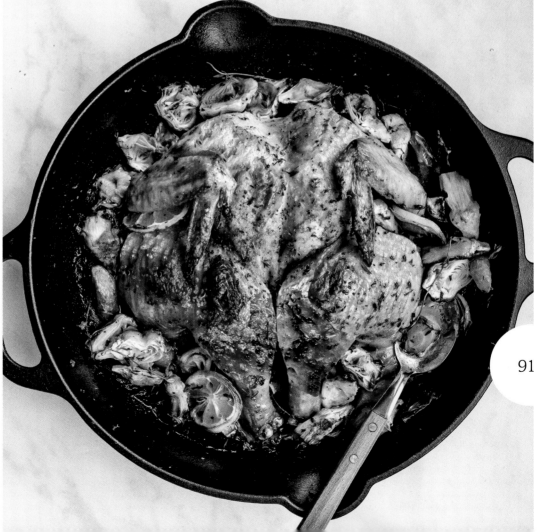

91

INTRODUCTION

The way you feed your body has a lot to do with your health—and your gut is the root of it all. Every cell, tissue, and organ depends on the body's digestive system to provide the nutrients it needs to keep functioning. But in today's world, we are constantly bombarded by chemicals, processed foods, additives, and toxins. This exposure accumulates in our bodies and contributes to inflammation and leads to disease. The sugar-filled Standard American Diet, over-the-counter and prescription medications, exhaustion, and chronic stress are constantly challenging how our bodies work and how our digestive systems function for optimal health.

A healthy gut is an integral part of overall health, but adopting new eating styles to support your gut can feel like a far stretch. You may be asking: Do I need to be gluten-free? How do I substitute for my many food sensitivities? What exactly is bone broth? Where do I get bones from?

It can be a lot to take in all at once. And when we are trying new things and searching for answers—all while symptoms or illnesses are holding us back—who wouldn't be tempted to reach for a quick fix? In the long run though, healing your gut and caring for your body is an ongoing lifestyle, and learning how to make this work is imperative to your success, health, and happiness. That's where I come in.

As a nutritional therapy practitioner and passionate, self-taught home chef, I believe healing your body with real food can be a stress-free lifestyle, filled with joy and flavor. No fuss and no fluff.

For me, cooking, meal prepping, eating more mindfully, practicing self-care, and honoring my bio-individuality have all become second nature to me. And I'm doing this while feeding a family, too! Making these practices a regular routine is one of the biggest reasons I've succeeded at managing my illnesses and putting them into remission.

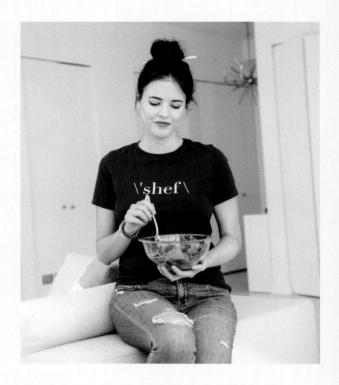

But it wasn't always this easy. I didn't suddenly eat more intuitively, or know how to sub dairy in a dish I was craving, or instantly see progress with my many digestive symptoms and inflammation. It wasn't carefree to navigate eating choices in social situations or at holidays or while traveling. At first, it was overwhelming, isolating, and stressful!

I've dealt with chronic health conditions for as long as I can remember. I thought it was my family's destiny to struggle with autoimmune diseases and chronic illness. It's all about our genes, right? I tried fad diets and intense cardio classes, but they only left me exhausted. When I should have been in the prime of my newly married and young professional life, my symptoms worsened instead of getting better. My body was crying out for help, yet I felt it was betraying me.

After being diagnosed with polycystic ovary syndrome (PCOS) and the autoimmune disease Hashimoto's thyroiditis by naturopaths and functional medical doctors, my healing journey began. After much education, practice, and experience, I went from fumbling around in the kitchen to being a confident home cook and holistic nutrition professional. I found creative ways to re-create beloved recipes such as Puerto Rican Pastelón (page 106) and Greek Spaghetti Squash Pastitsio (page 108), as well as restaurant favorites like Chicken Pad Thai with Green Papaya Noodles (page 147). I put my illnesses into remission, and I had a healthy pregnancy and baby girl (which I thought wouldn't be possible for me). Through all of this, I've gained a new respect and love for my body.

Many of us live fearful of getting diagnosed with one of the dreaded, yet commonplace, diseases: diabetes, Alzheimer's, heart disease, cancer, autoimmune disease. We know that diet and lifestyle play a role, but we worry our fate may lie in "bad genes," and we may feel we have no control over our health. That's simply untrue, and many of our choices come down to our day-to-day routines, what we put in our mouths, and how we live. The science of epigenetics backs this up: Genes can be "turned on" or "off." Our fate isn't predetermined.

Wherever you are in your health and healing journey, whatever brought you to this book, know that you can take control of your health. Over the years, I've helped hundreds of clients and inspired millions of readers on my food and wellness blog, *Food by Mars* (www.foodbymars.com). The gut-healthy lifestyle I share with you in this book includes the tools I've used on myself and with my clients. I will be lovingly blunt with you along the way—as a New Yorker, that's the only way I know how!

Your body wants to heal, and it is always working to bring you back to equilibrium. By recruiting both the dietary and lifestyle aspects of the Paleo template, you'll learn so much about your body and how to listen to its signals, eating in a more mindful and intuitive state to provide what your body needs in the present. That's the real power here, to cut through the noise and get back in tune with your body and your health.

This information helped me find joy, ease, and confidence in the way I nourish myself day in and day out. And I want that for you, too! I've learned healing isn't linear. It's messy. And it can be beautiful, delicious, and transformative. I'm so happy you're here, and it's my pleasure to support your journey as you listen to your body and adopt this new, healing lifestyle!

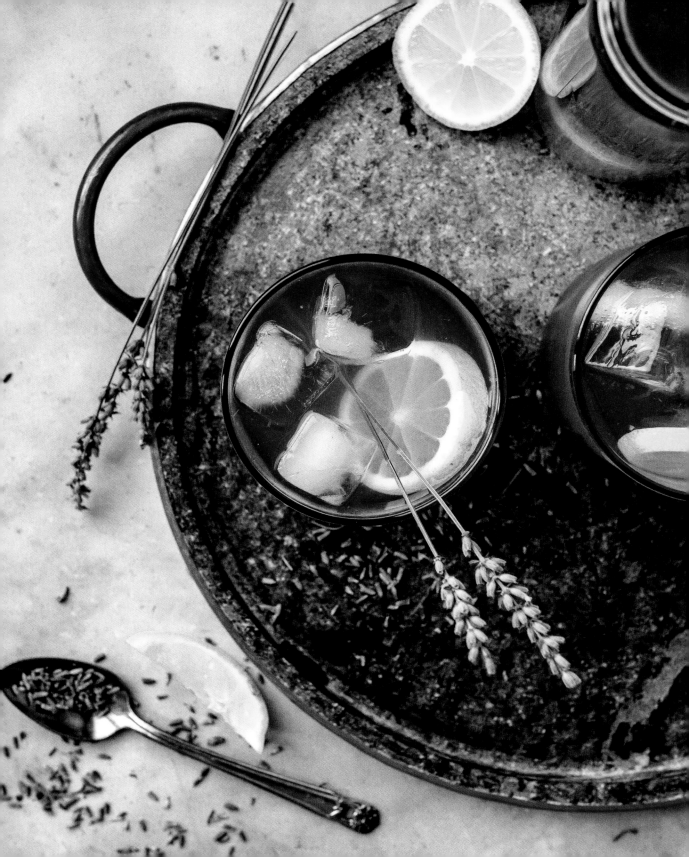

1

GUT HEALING WITH PALEO

Many of us eat while driving, watching TV, scrolling social media, or working through our lunch breaks. This means our digestion is off to a poor start. We also put up with common symptoms of bloating, abdominal discomfort, and irregularity, eventually leading to more serious chronic conditions such as acid reflux, heartburn, indigestion, GERD, and IBS. But we don't have to!

Turning it all around begins in the *brain*. This chapter walks you through the digestive process because knowledge is power. Then we'll cover the basics of the Paleo and Autoimmune Protocol (AIP) diets and the benefits they can offer as you take the reins on your health. Chapter 2 will help you know exactly how to support your gut health in your everyday life, because you're in this for the long haul, baby. I'll show you how!

The Gut-Brain Connection

Contrary to what you might have thought, digestion doesn't start in your stomach or even your mouth. It all begins in the brain. You need your nervous system to be in a parasympathetic state, what's often referred to, quite perfectly, as the "rest and digest" state. This is because digestion takes up a ton of power and our body has to be ready for it. Your brain needs to signal to your mouth (to salivate), to your stomach (to create strong hydrochloric acid), to your pancreas (to create juices and enzymes), to your gallbladder (to create bile), so on and so forth.

Chewing is essential to good digestion and nutrient absorption. It also helps to stimulate more saliva production. Saliva helps to break down the foods, specifically carbohydrates. Chewing your food thoroughly and savoring your food helps to slow you down and let your body do its work.

Ways to Promote Strong Stomach Acid

→ Eat in a parasympathetic state (page 24) and manage stress (page 38).
→ Reduce sugar.
→ Start your day with warm lemon water.
→ Try 1 teaspoon of apple cider vinegar in water before your meals.
→ Consider supplementing with betaine HCl. (This won't be right for everyone and dosage will vary to each individual. Consult a practitioner.)

The food you've chewed up is passed down the esophagus and poured into the stomach. Gastric juices help break down the food further. While acidity in the body isn't welcome elsewhere, it's crucial inside the stomach. Hydrochloric acid in your stomach triggers production of an enzyme called pepsin, which breaks down proteins into amino acids (aka the building blocks of our bodies). The acid also acts as a disinfectant to kill any pathogens you might have consumed in the food; this is a line of defense against food poisoning.

After the stomach has its turn with the food breakdown, the food is now released slowly into the first part of the small intestine (the duodenum), where the fats signal the release of bile from the gallbladder (which is where the liver stores the bile), which then helps with the digestion and emulsification of the fats. The pancreas releases more enzymes that help with the digestion of fat, protein, and carbohydrates. To help this stage of digestion, support your liver with regular movement, sweating, and staying well-hydrated. Be careful not to overconsume caffeine or alcohol, which put more of a load on the liver. Eating healthy fats also ensures you are using the bile stored in the gallbladder and it can be used efficiently for digestion.

Along the walls of the intestine there is a mucosal layer with villi and microvilli (I like to picture them as bristles on a toothbrush). A healthy gut lining will have tight junctions: Picture a brand-new toothbrush with tight bristles versus a six-month-old beat-up toothbrush with loose bristles. Tight junctions can be compromised, or become "leaky," when affected by inflammation, stress, or pathogens. This is called "leaky gut" or intestinal permeability. And, because roughly 70 to 80 percent of our immune cells are in this area, the health of the small intestine is essential.

The large intestine, or colon, is where elimination (a bowel movement) will occur. Various bacterial strains reside in the colon, including 100 billion to 100 trillion symbiotic organisms! They help to ferment dietary fibers into short-chain fatty acids, which are a source of energy that directly nourishes the cells that line the colon. They produce B vitamins and vitamin K. They also metabolize bile acids and produce important proteins.

What Is Leaky Gut?

Also known as intestinal permeability, "leaky gut" is a condition where the villi and microvilli of the gut lining have been compromised or damaged to the point of allowing food particles to leak out into the bloodstream.

Common Symptoms of Leaky Gut
→ Food sensitivities
→ Inflammation
→ Chronic diarrhea, constipation, or bloating
→ Nutritional deficiencies
→ Fatigue
→ Headaches
→ Brain fog
→ Skin problems, such as acne, rashes, or eczema
→ Joint pain

In recent years, health care practitioners have found that healing intestinal permeability is fundamental to overall health, and this requires lifestyle changes beyond the healing phase. When we use a nutritional therapy–based strategy for improving gut health—food as medicine—we also need to integrate it into an everyday holistic lifestyle.

What Is the Connection between the Brain and the Gut?

The brain is connected to the gut by the vagus nerve. It runs from the brain stem to part of the colon, and it oversees a vast array of crucial bodily functions including mood, immune response, digestion, and heart rate. This connection represents the main component of the parasympathetic nervous system, also known as the "rest and digest" state that needs to be activated for proper digestion.

The digestive system also has its own nervous system, the enteric nervous system (ENS), consisting of approximately 100 million nerve cells in and around the gastrointestinal (GI) tract. The ENS receives inputs from the sympathetic and parasympathetic nervous systems, but it can also function independently of them. Emeran Mayer, M.D., author of *The Mind-Gut Connection*, compares the ENS to a local government, like the mayor of a city that can run routine functions independently of the federal government (the emotional brain center). But when there's a federal emergency like stress or trauma, the emotional brain, or federal government in this analogy, will divert the "local government agency," or the ENS, from its normal routines. The digestive system will switch back to local control once the emotion or scenario is managed and passes.

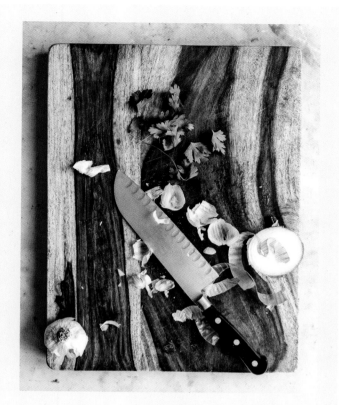

The ENS is also intimately interconnected with millions of immune cells. These cells survey the digestive system and convey information, such as whether the stomach is bloated or whether there's an infection in the GI tract or insufficient blood flow back to the brain. Thus, the brain and GI system communicate with each other in both directions: The mayor communicates up the chain to the federal government to report back on what's happening in their city.

The gut and brain are interconnected and constantly in communication in both directions. The state of one affects the other, and affects other functions such as digestion, blood sugar regulation, and immune response. If you're supporting this connection daily on all fronts, you're supporting a keystone to your greater health and well-being.

What Is the Paleo Diet?

Today, millions of people in the United States suffer from chronic disorders, including 25 million who have irritable bowel syndrome (IBS) and between 23.5 and 50 million who suffer from autoimmune diseases. And now you can see why—there's an enormous disconnect between our modern lifestyles and diet with how our digestive system is actually meant to work. Returning to a more natural, anti-inflammatory diet can help turn it all around.

The Paleo template maximizes foods that support healing and minimizes foods that may cause harm to the body. This shift in diet lays the groundwork for a healthy digestive system and a diverse, robust microbiome. The focus is on prebiotic and probiotic foods, a variety of vegetables, fruits, and other whole plant foods (providing quality dietary fiber), and a variety of animal proteins.

While some of the Paleo principles may feel new (or new to you), they might seem more familiar to your grandparents—or more likely, your great-grandparents. Paleo principles are more traditional to the way many cultures lived before modern technology, processed foods, refined sugar, and mainstream inaccurate "dietary guidelines" led us astray from our body's innate wisdom.

The Paleo guidelines are not "law" or gospel. They're a comprehensive template to use while tuning in to your body's own needs. It's about food and about lifestyle, as all pieces work synergistically together.

The Paleo diet eliminates foods with little nutritional value as well as foods that may be difficult to digest and/or may cause inflammation. Paleo emphasizes whole foods, with two-thirds or more of your plate covered with plant foods. The other third is animal protein, which has vital nutrients and essential amino acids that can be found only in animal products. The quality and sourcing of animal products is important to the diet for both nutritional and ethical reasons, and you'll often see meat represented as a central topic of the Paleo diet—but that doesn't make it a meat-only diet by any means.

Paleo Template Basics

Eat real food. Focus on nutrient-dense, properly prepared whole food. See page 27 for more details.

Move your body. Enjoy your favorite form of exercise. Try a standing desk. Take walking breaks. Make dance, play, and movement a part of daily life.

Connect with others. Humans thrive on connection. Spend time engaging with loved ones and friends, being present in their company.

Sleep well. Our hormones and circadian rhythm require us to be active in the daytime and restful at night. We need seven to nine hours of quality sleep at night to relax and restore.

Get outside. We need vitamin D from the sun's rays, and we need to breathe in fresh air while connecting with nature. Make the effort to schedule daily outside time.

Unplug. Logging out of social media, limiting screen time, and cutting out other external noise helps us to spend time with ourselves and tune in.

Connect with yourself. Practice self-care by meditating, journaling, or finding quiet, simple time alone. Make recharging yourself and reducing stress a daily ritual—even a few minutes throughout the day can make a difference.

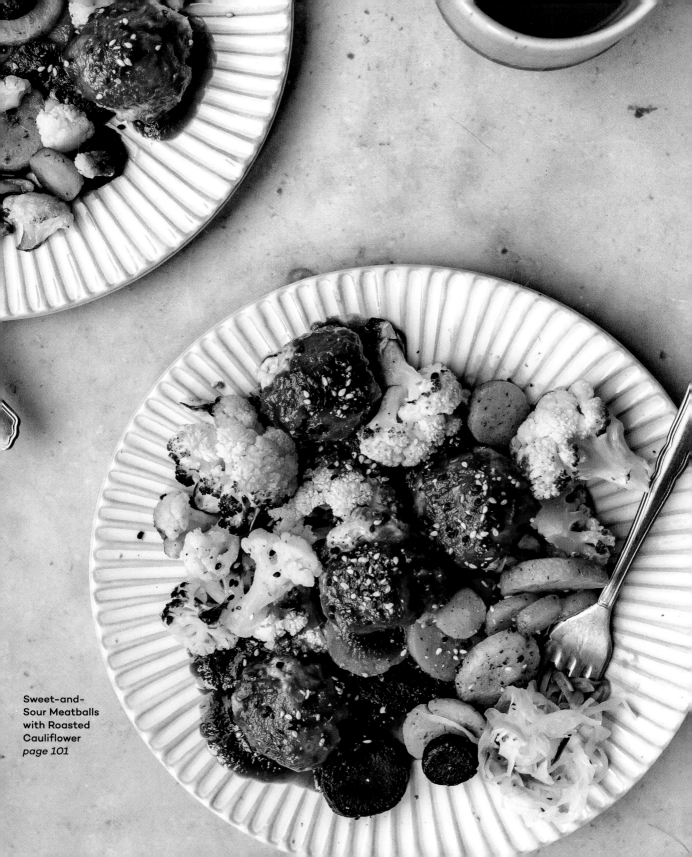

Sweet-and-Sour Meatballs with Roasted Cauliflower
page 101

PALEO GUIDELINES: *Foods to Enjoy*

Cruciferous vegetables
arugula, bok choy, broccoli, broccoli rabe (rapini), Brussels sprouts, cabbage, cauliflower, collard greens, daikon, kale (all varieties), kohlrabi, radishes, rutabaga, turnips, watercress

Root vegetables
acorn squash, arrowroot, beets, burdock, butternut squash, carrot, celeriac, delicata squash, ginger, Jerusalem artichoke (sunchoke), jicama, kabocha squash, parsnip, pumpkin, spaghetti squash, winter squash (all varieties), sweet potato, taro, tiger nut, water chestnut, yacón, yam, yucca (cassava, manioc, tapioca)

Leafy greens
amaranth greens, beet greens, carrot tops, celery, chicory, cress, dandelion greens, endive, fiddlehead, land cress, lettuce (all types), pea leaves, pumpkin sprouts, purslane, radicchio, radish sprouts, spinach, squash blossoms, sweet potato greens, Swiss chard, water spinach

Sea vegetables
dulse, kombu, nori, sea kale, sea lettuce, wakame

Mushrooms and edible fungi
button (including portobello and cremini), chanterelle, king trumpet, lion's mane, maitake, matsutake, morel, oyster, shiitake, truffle, winter; yeast (baker's, brewer's, nutritional)

Fruits
all berries such as acai, blueberry, cranberry, elderberry, mulberry, muscadine grape, raspberry, sea buckthorn, strawberry; apples, apricot, artichoke, asparagus, banana, camu camu, cantaloupe, capers, celery, cherry, coconut, date, dragon fruit, edible flowers, fennel, fig, honeydew, jackfruit, kiwi, kumquat, lychee, mango, melon pear, nectarine, okra, papaya, passionfruit, peach, pear, pepino melon, Persian melon, persimmon, pineapple, plantain, plum, pomegranate, quince, rhubarb, soursop, squash blossoms, star fruit, watermelon, zucchini; citrus fruits such as citron, clementine, grapefruit, key lime, lemon, lime, mandarin, Meyer lemon, orange, tangerine, yuzu

Alliums (or aromatics) and herbs
chives, garlic, leek, onion, pearl onion, ramps, scallion, shallot, spring onion; basil leaves, chamomile, chervil, cilantro, curry leaves, dill weed, fenugreek leaves, lavender, lemongrass, marjoram, oregano, parsley, peppermint, rosemary, sage, savory, spearmint, tarragon, thyme

Spices
allspice, anise, annatto seed, black caraway, black pepper, caraway, cardamom, celery seed, cinnamon, cloves, coriander seed, cumin seed, dill seed, fennel seed, fenugreek seed, garlic, ginger, green peppercorns, juniper, mace, mustard seed, nutmeg, pink peppercorns, saffron, star anise, sumac, truffles, turmeric, vanilla bean, wasabi, white pepper

Wild fish, seafood, and shellfish
anchovy, arctic char, bass, bream, carp, catfish, cod, eel, haddock, halibut, herring, mackerel, mahi-mahi, monkfish, mullet, pollock, salmon, sardine, snapper, sole, swordfish, tilapia, tilefish, trout, tuna; caviar/roe, clam, conch, crab, crawfish, cuttlefish, lobster, mussel, octopus, oyster, prawn, scallop, shrimp, snail, squid

Red meat
beef, bison/buffalo, boar, deer, elk, goat, hare, lamb, moose, mutton, pork, rabbit

Poultry and eggs
chicken, duck, eggs (chicken, duck, goose, quail), goose, guinea hen, ostrich, partridge, pheasant, quail, turkey

Offal
bone broth, bone marrow, fats and other trimmings such as tallow and lard, cheek and jowl meat, heart, kidney, liver, rinds (skin), sweetbreads, tripe

High-fat fruits
avocado, olives (green and black)

Animal fats (ideally from grass-fed or pasture-raised animals)
bacon fat, lard, leaf lard, poultry fat, schmaltz, tallow, pan drippings

Plant oils (ideally all cold-pressed, unrefined, organic, and ethically sourced)
avocado oil, coconut oil, extra-virgin olive oil, macadamia nut oil, palm oil, palm shortening, red palm oil, sesame oil, toasted sesame oil, walnut oil

Nuts
almonds, baruka nuts, Brazil nuts, cashews, chestnuts, coconut, hazelnuts (filberts), macadamia nuts, pecans, pili nuts, pine nuts, pistachios, walnuts

Seeds
cacao (chocolate), chia, flax, hemp, poppy, pumpkin (pepitas), sacha inchi, sesame, sunflower

Probiotic and fermented foods beet and other types of kvasses, coconut milk kefir or Instant Pot Coconut Yogurt (page 187), kombucha, lacto-fermented relishes and salsas, sauerkraut, kimchi, pickles, Fermented Coleslaw (page 184), water kefir

PALEO GUIDELINES: *Foods to Avoid*

→ **Processed foods and additives:** synthetic food dyes; certain preservatives, emulsifiers, thickeners, and stabilizers that can cause inflammation

→ **Refined sugar:** brown sugar, corn syrup, granulated sugar, and other names for sugar such as fructose, dextrin, glucose, inulin, and malt syrup

→ **Legumes and soy (legumes with edible pods such as green beans and peas are fine):** all beans including kidney beans and black beans, chickpeas, peanuts, pulses such as lentils

→ **Gluten, grains, and pseudograins:** buckwheat, einkorn, emmer, millet, quinoa, rice, rye, spelt, teff, wheat

→ **Dairy (especially conventional):** cheese, cream, half-and-half, milk

→ **Refined and processed seed oils:** canola oil, corn oil, safflower oil, soybean oil, vegetable oil

→ **Excessive alcohol (wine, beer, cocktails):** Alcohol in moderation and if able to, low-sugar, organic, or biodynamic wine is recommended.

A Typical Home-Cooked Paleo Plate

→ 4 to 8 ounces of high-quality animal protein (around 30 grams of protein)

→ 2 or more servings of nonstarchy vegetables (such as cruciferous veggies; think greens)

→ 1 serving of a "slow" carb (e.g., starchy vegetables such as sweet potato or winter squash)

→ Fresh or dried herbs, nuts/seeds, and spices to add more flavor and nutrients

→ Everything cooked or dressed with healthy fats (such as extra-virgin olive oil, animal fat like lard, or ghee)

→ A small cup of filtered water

→ And, for extra gut love, a cup of bone broth or forkful of fermented foods

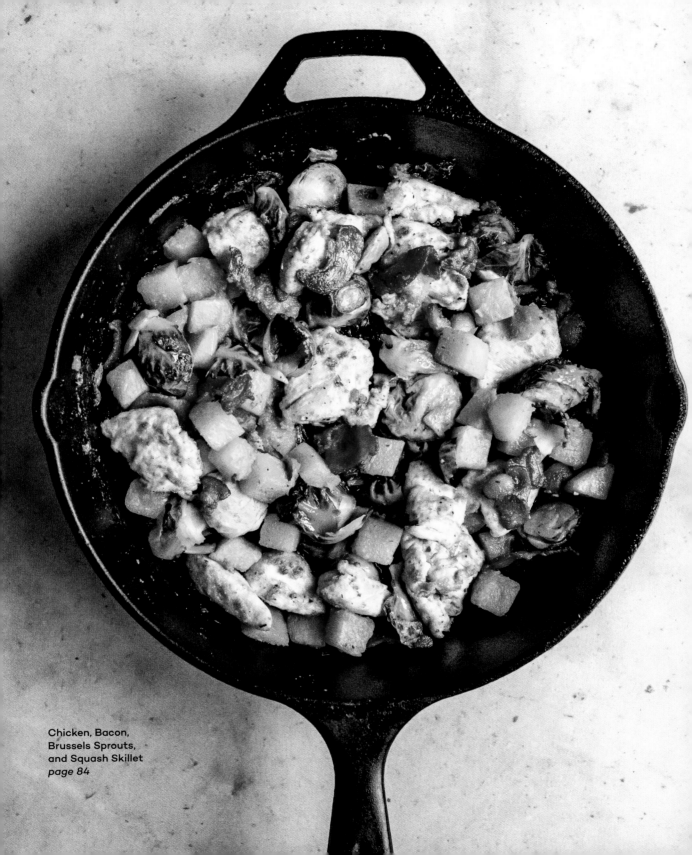

Chicken, Bacon,
Brussels Sprouts,
and Squash Skillet
page 84

What Is the Autoimmune Protocol Diet?

The Autoimmune Protocol (AIP) diet provides more specific food restrictions beyond the Paleo template. This diet can be very supportive to those with an autoimmune disease or chronic digestive conditions. When planning to try it, I'd suggest using it after using the Paleo template first for at least 30 days. It starts with a short-term food elimination phase, followed by a four-stage reintroduction phase. The diet emphasizes nutrient-dense healing foods, such as broths and organ meats, to help heal the gut so you may reintroduce foods back safely based on your physiology and healing stage.

Before you begin AIP, ensure you are practicing self-care and feel ready for the entire process: Some people find they feel so much better with the eliminations that they want to stay on the elimination phase for several months or even years! Keep in mind that only focusing on eliminations may leave you feeling restricted and hangry, and can cause deficiencies in key nutrients. A diversity of foods is *crucial* to your gut health and healing. I recommend planning out the elimination time frame, with a commitment to going through the four-stage reintroductions in an organized way. It's helpful to have the support of a practitioner such as a nutritional therapy practitioner or certified AIP coach.

By applying the Paleo template and AIP, you learn lessons about food and how it affects your health and well-being. During the reintroduction stage, you might find foods on the "avoid" Paleo food list that are fine for you! Many people enjoy properly prepared beans, rice, or quality grass-fed dairy in moderation with ease, especially after giving their gut a break to heal and to handle these foods better. Just remember that there is no "one size fits all" approach to nutrition. Everyone's journey will look different, and everyone's path toward balance is unique and subject to change.

The Benefits of Paleo and AIP

These diets improve health by restoring balance to the body through eliminations and food choices. Clinical trials show that a Paleo diet improves cardiovascular disease risk factors, reduces inflammation, improves glucose tolerance, and helps with weight loss and metabolism. It can even improve autoimmune disease (for more details, see Dr. Sarah Ballantyne's *Paleo Principles*). Think of Paleo as a foundation and AIP as further guidelines geared specifically to those with autoimmune disease, digestive disorders, and chronic illness.

The real underlying beauty of the Paleo template is that it can restore your body back to balance while helping you personalize your diet to your bio-individuality. When we can strengthen our digestion, balance our blood sugar, and support natural detoxification, we are much better equipped to listen to our bodies. And this liberates you from having to strictly or blindly follow a diet. When used as it is intended, consider Paleo as a path back to nature so you can always find the answers for yourself and support your health at the root.

New to the AIP diet?

When considering trying the AIP diet: I'd suggest using it after first using the Paleo template for at least thirty days. AIP starts with a short-term food elimination phase, followed by a four-stage reintroduction phase which is generally outlined in this book, and recipes are marked with AIP notes and substitutions for those on AIP or with sensitivities to nuts, seeds, eggs, or nightshades for example. However, it's recommended to be well-prepared and supported when embarking on AIP if this is new to you and something you'd like to use on your chronic illness healing journey.

AIP GUIDELINES:
Eliminations

In addition to following the Paleo template, which is gluten-, grain-, soy-, legume-, and dairy-free, these foods are eliminated during the elimination phase of AIP (for one to three months before reintroductions). Updates are sometimes made to these lists, so you can always stay up to date or see more elaborated lists by following the work of Dr. Sarah Ballantyne and AutoimmuneWellness.com.

→ Nightshades (foods and spices), including tomatoes, tomatillos, white potatoes, all peppers, eggplants, goji berries, ashwagandha, tobacco

→ Certain spices (fruit- and seed-based), including allspice, anise, annatto, canola, caraway, cardamom, celery seed, coriander, cumin, fennel seed, fenugreek, juniper, mustard, nutmeg, paprika, pepper, sumac

→ Certain vegetable oils, including canola, corn, ghee, safflower, soybean, and vegetable

→ Coffee

→ Chocolate/cacao

→ Eggs

→ Nuts and seeds

→ Alcohol

→ Food additives, such as refined or added sugars and sugar alcohols

→ Algae: spirulina and chlorella

Common Symptoms of Nightshade Sensitivity

→ Joint pain
→ Stiffness upon waking, or stiffness after sitting for longs periods of time
→ Muscle pain and tension
→ Muscle tremors
→ Poor healing
→ Insomnia
→ Skin rashes
→ Heartburn
→ Stomach pain and digestive difficulties
→ Headaches
→ Mood swings
→ Brain fog
→ Depression

AIP GUIDELINES: *Reintroductions*

Dr. Sarah Ballantyne has several resources on the AIP diet, including studies and trials on its effects. This is the recommended four-stage reintroduction schedule. You'll notice some non-Paleo foods like lentils and rice in later stages. Remember that both Paleo and AIP are templates to use as you uncover which foods work best for you and in what amounts. I recommend using a food/mood journal to track and going slow, staggering each food by a few days so you can truly feel it out.

STAGE 1
→ Egg yolks
→ Fruit-, berry-, and seed-based spices
→ Seed and nut oils
→ Ghee (grass-fed)
→ Occasional coffee
→ Cocoa or chocolate
→ Peas and legumes with edible pods (green beans, sugar snap peas, snow peas, etc.)
→ Legume sprouts

STAGE 2
→ Seeds
→ Nuts
→ Chia seeds
→ Coffee on a daily basis
→ Egg whites
→ Grass-fed butter
→ Alcohol in small quantities

STAGE 3
→ Eggplant
→ Sweet peppers
→ Paprika
→ Peeled white potatoes
→ Grass-fed dairy
→ Lentils, split peas, and chickpeas

STAGE 4
→ Chili peppers and nightshade spices
→ Tomatoes
→ Unpeeled potatoes
→ Alcohol in larger quantities
→ Gluten-free grains and pseudograins such as quinoa
→ Traditionally prepared (soaked/sprouted) or fermented legumes
→ White rice
→ Specific foods you are sensitive to

A Holistic Approach to Gut Healing

Removing Irritants and Allergens While Healing
Using the Paleo Diet Template (and possibly AIP when needed), you'll learn which eliminations benefit your body by going through the elimination exercise, crowding your plates with nutrient-dense healing foods, and discovering through trial and error what foods do best for your body based on your bio-individuality. Then you can take it from there using these diets as a starting point to get in tune (and not as gospel).

Minding the Gut-Brain Connection
It all begins in the brain, and taking care of your stress combined with mindful eating is a key, foundational strategy to support gut healing and maintaining your gut health over the long term. Nothing else you try will work well enough without this in place.

Repairing and Restoring Balance
Gut healing with Paleo means promoting strong stomach acid with food and lifestyle supports, considering supplements like betaine HCl and/or digestive enzymes, using soothing herbs such as aloe vera and marshmallow root to help heal inflammation, and improving the gut wall integrity with L-glutamine and other amino acids abundantly found in bone broth and animal products.

Repopulating and Supporting the Microbiome
By eating prebiotics and fermented foods, and possibly trying probiotic supplements, we reinoculate the microbiome. Don't forget bio-individuality and having a plan for reintroducing nutritious whole foods throughout the healing process and especially as you see results!

Now, we need to consider the everyday, beautiful, messy life that exists no matter what stage of healing you're in. There are pivotal lifestyle and diet practices to help you succeed with maintaining your gut health, which we'll cover next.

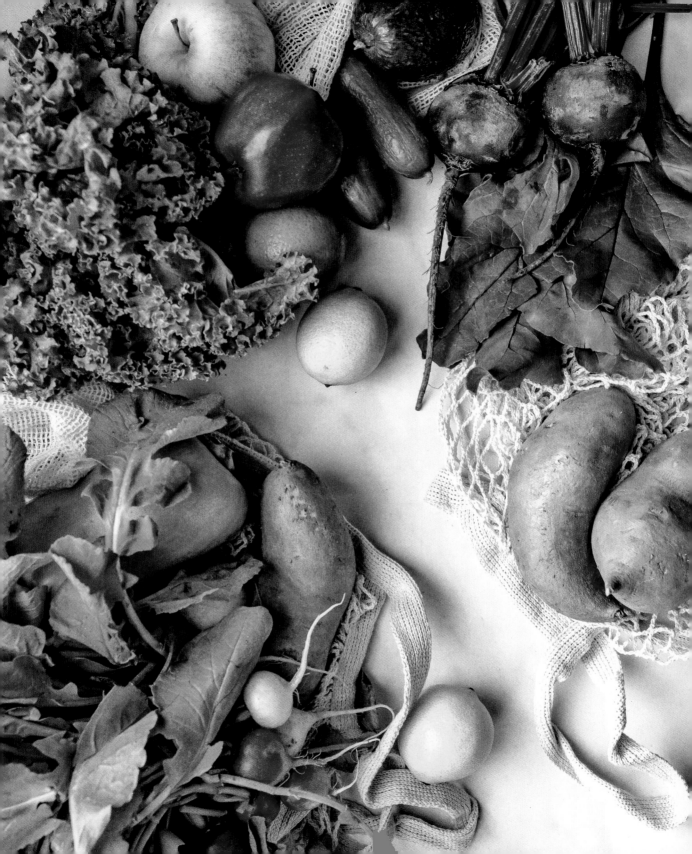

2

10 EVERYDAY PRACTICES FOR OPTIMAL DIGESTION

Gut healing is not a one-shot deal. It's not just about what you eat, but *how* and *why* you eat it. It's about building lifestyle habits, slowly and over time. While that might sound boring . . . that's what actually works! I promised I'd always be lovingly blunt, didn't I?

Lifestyle changes may seem challenging when adopting a new way of eating, but it can be a fun and joyful experience when you're open to trying new things and getting creative in the kitchen. Gut healing is a beautiful lifelong practice, and you can see remarkable results by adopting a "progress over perfection" mindset. Listen to your body and add a few simple practices to your daily life to strengthen your digestive system, support your immune system, and balance your blood sugar (and thus, your hormones and energy). Most of these habits will make you feel better all day, every day!

#1 Mindful Eating

Mindfulness is the act of paying attention to what's happening right in front of you in the present. It's about being aware of what you're doing and simply observing without judgment. It's living in the now, without distractions such as internal mind chatter, devices, or multitasking.

Mindful eating is the practice of slowing down and being present as you eat. It supports your digestion in the moment, improves overall gut health, and encourages a healthy relationship with food and your body. A parasympathetic state is required for proper digestion and it begins in the brain. This is why mindful eating isn't just a "nice thing to practice." It's actually crucial to your ability to kick off digestion properly.

It's common to confuse physical hunger pangs and normal stomach sensations with feelings of anxiety, nervousness, or stress. You may crave snacks or want to chew something. You may describe yourself as a "stress eater." Or you may go in the opposite direction and lose your appetite when under stress. Mindful eating can help you realize a pattern here and work to feed your body when you're truly hungry. The practice can also help you avoid stress eating or skipping meals, which will both compromise digestion.

Mindful Eating Basics

The basics are simple, but take consistent practice. There's no prize for perfection here, just little by little habit-building. First, assess your hunger. Check in with your gut and how you're feeling. Ask yourself, "Am I physically hungry?" A physical hunger should feel like hunger pangs or sensations in the stomach of gurgling, growling, and feeling empty. If you're feeling irritable, cranky, or "hangry," you likely haven't eaten enough throughout the day or are very dehydrated.

When it is time to eat, ground yourself in the present moment. This activates a relaxation response in the body. It's like signaling to the body "I'm safe" so it can flip the switch to being in the parasympathetic state needed to start the digestive process.

Put distractions away.
Be seated. Toss the phone or shut off the TV so you can be present and pay attention to what's in front of you.

Slow down and breathe.
Take three to five deep belly breaths before your first bite. These should be deep breaths into the belly, fully inhaling and exhaling.

Be present in the moment.
Look at your food and the company you are with, or even say a form of "grace" silently or aloud if you'd like.

Chew your food thoroughly and savor each bite.
If this is sounding too simple, it's because it should be! But this is usually the biggest issue with modern-day eating habits. We eat quickly while stressed or preoccupied. We forget to chew our food!

Pause mid-meal and check in with yourself.
It's so easy to slip back into old habits, and that's why this is a practice. Now is the time to reset if you need to. When the plate is half empty, ask yourself: Am I still eating slowly? Have I wandered off to grab my mobile device or gotten up to multitask? Can I bring my attention back to the meal, to the flavors, to chewing, to breathing completely? Am I still hungry or am I feeling more satiated?

Finish your meal when you're just about full.
It takes approximately twenty minutes for fullness to register. That's why checking in and ending a little bit sooner will help prevent feelings of sickness or discomfort. And if you find you are still hungry, go back for more! This isn't about depriving yourself. It's about reconnecting and tuning in to the hunger and satiation cues from your body.

Chewing Challenge

→ Cut food up on your plate as you would for a toddler! This will automatically get smaller bites into your mouth and slow you down.
→ Put your fork or spoon down between bites to allow yourself to fully enjoy each bite.
→ When chewing, notice the flavors, savor each dimension of flavor as you taste it, and silently remark on them. Is the food tasting sweeter? Earthier? Is it soft, chewy, crispy?
→ Just when you think you can't chew any longer, add three more chews just for good measure and finally swallow. (Somewhere around applesauce consistency is a great target!)

Oral Health and Gut Health

Keeping your mouth clean and healthy is also paramount to your gut health. Brush your teeth two to three times per day. Flossing and tongue scraping clean out bacteria more deeply to support your digestive system.

Your Own Personal Mindful Eating Practice

Make mealtime sacred and set boundaries.
Set breaks for your meals throughout the day and honor that time to be fully present. This could mean adding "lunch break" to your calendar, setting an alarm ten minutes earlier so you can have a proper sit-down breakfast, and clearing the table for dinner to make sure it's unrushed and pleasurable.

Cook most of your food at home.
Connecting with your food starts long before you sit down to a plate of food. The sourcing, shopping, cooking, and preparing of the meal gets you connected to the food in a deeper way. And, if someone else cooked it for you at home or at a restaurant, take extra time to be grateful to the chef and the sources of the meal.

Make it a sensual experience.
Use your five senses when you eat: Look at your food. Touch it and smell it. Hear yourself chew it, and slow down to really taste it. Engage your senses by buying a new lunch bag or container for workdays; use a beautiful bowl or plate your meal with fresh herbs as a garnish at home. Try lighting a candle at your dinner table and dimming the lights with some soft music! Do whatever elevates the experience to make it more pleasurable, using touch, sight, hearing, smell, and taste. It can be so simple but so impactful. Have fun with it!

Show respect for yourself and your practice.
This won't be an overnight change, and some days it'll feel easier than others. Show compassion for yourself to let go of judgment and to keep going. Being present and practicing mindfulness is a moment-to-moment decision, and those little decisions add up to great transformation. Don't stop because of a stressful day, week, or month—mindfulness is always there waiting for you.

#2 Fasting

At its most basic, fasting just means not eating. It can be a powerful tool for supporting your gut health, metabolism, blood sugar regulation, weight management, and neurological health. The duration is up to you, and you must listen to your body as you try it. Factors such as health conditions, stress, sleep quality, and weight (especially if underweight) all need to be considered.

When setting a time range for when you eat and when you don't, the key indicators to notice are your energy, sleep, mood, stress, hunger, satiation, digestion, and elimination. You'll want to monitor yourself closely and give it a good amount of time to see how fasting is affecting you. Try it and see if you notice changes in your digestion and overall sense of well-being. (If it's causing more stress on your life, table it.)

Getting Started

Here's an easy way to begin a "14:10" fast. You've likely done this before or do it regularly without even realizing it.

→ Fast for at least fourteen hours overnight (from dinner to breakfast and stay hydrated with water).
→ Eat balanced meals throughout the day. (See pg. 17 for a typical home cooked meal template.)
→ Allow for three to four hours of rest between meals with regular hydration.

Eating this way aligns with your circadian rhythm, which coincides with your natural sleep/wake cycles. This "body clock" is important to regulating blood sugar, and thus your overall energy and hormones. Your ability to digest usually peaks at midday and then decreases from there. To maximize this natural rhythm, have your larger meals during the day and a smaller dinner in the early evening.

Personalizing Your Eating Schedule

It's best to give a 14:10 fast a two-week trial and assess its effects. Journal how you're feeling and how your body is reacting. This will help you see if something has worked or not, and you can rely on listening to your body versus blindly following diet advice. The greatest value in trying these practices is getting more in tune with your own body. Learn what works *for you*, and honor it above all else. Be sure to pay attention to how fasting fits within your life schedule and routines. Shift workers, caregivers, and those working a lot of hours can sometimes find tweaking schedules to be challenging. Take time to look for ways to set boundaries or get support for your trial fast. You can even work up to a fast by making step-by-step changes, integrating this over time. For example, start by switching the time of one meal. Tackle that for at least one week, then look at break times between meals and adjust those. The key is to set yourself up for success!

As you explore rhythmic eating, have fun with it. Seriously. You're on a journey, and it's important to show yourself a lot of self-compassion. Treat your body, health, and healing journey as you would treat caring for a child or a sick loved one. Let go of impatience and perfectionism, and give yourself all the patience, love, and openness you deserve.

Allow the Digestive System to Rest

Fasting is about timing, but it's also focused on giving your body an opportunity to rest. Constant snacking in the absence of true physical hunger inundates the body with more work to do. And when you are snacking while rushed, on the go, or in front of a screen mindlessly, you aren't even signaling to your body that it's time to digest.

If you're hungry, snack mindfully. If you're not, skip it. If stress or emotions push you to snack, call it out, recognize what's true hunger and what's not, and satisfy your need elsewhere with self-care.

So, what are you doing between meals then? Be active or rest, depending on what your body needs. And be sure to hydrate! Remember: Drinking during a meal can squelch stomach acid, which needs to be strong during meals. So, sip what you need during meals and get the bulk of your water between meals. Warm or room temperature water is ideal to keep you regular and keep digestion moving.

#3 Eating Quality Food

The Paleo template focuses on nutrient-dense whole foods over nutrient-less processed food. After all, if you read a food label and can't understand half the ingredients, why would your gut be able to make sense of it? We begin by removing irritants, refined sugars, processed and artificial additives, gluten, conventional dairy, and soy, while enjoying whole fruits and vegetables, well-sourced animal protein, and quality fats.

Sourcing Nutrient-Dense Food

It can be confusing to know what the best sources of food are. Is organic best? Or grass-fed or natural? I've outlined your options so you can make the best decision based on what's available to you. (Source: nourishedkitchen.com)

MEATS

Best: Wild game; local grass-fed AND grass-finished beef, bison, and lamb; pasture-raised pork
Better: Nonlocal grass-finished and pasture-raised meats
Good: Organic, raised without antibiotics
⊘ **Limit or Avoid:** Meat raised from animals in conventional "factory farms" that are treated with growth hormones, drugs, and routine antibiotics

POULTRY & EGGS

Best: Wild birds; local pasture-raised poultry; eggs purchased directly from the farmer (preferably soy-free and GMO-free)
Better: Pasture-raised poultry and eggs from a local or online grocery shop
Good: Organic eggs; high omega-3 eggs; meat from "free-range" chickens and turkeys
⊘ **Limit or Avoid:** Conventionally raised poultry and eggs from farms that cage the animals or do not allow access to outdoors and free movement

FISH & SEAFOOD

Best: Sustainably wild-caught fish with low mercury levels such as salmon, sardines, and anchovies; wild-caught shrimp from sustainable fisheries; and shellfish such as oysters, mussels, and clams that are sustainably farmed in clean waters
Better: Sustainably wild-caught fish with lower mercury levels such as skipjack tuna
Good: Wild-caught fish with moderately high mercury content such as halibut, albacore tuna, and sablefish; sustainable farmed fish
⊘ **Limit or Avoid:** Fish high in mercury content such as king mackerel, blue fish, orange roughy, grouper, shark, and ahi tuna and farmed fish (unless sustainably farmed)

FRUITS & VEGETABLES

Best: Fresh local, organic, or biodynamic fruits and vegetables
Better: Fresh and frozen organic fruits and vegetables
Good: Fresh and/or local conventionally grown fruits and vegetables with low pesticide residue (refer to the Environmental Working Group's Dirty Dozen and Clean 15 lists, found on their website: www.EWG.org)
⊘ **Limit or Avoid:** Conventionally grown fruits and vegetables on the EWG's Dirty Dozen list that indicate a high pesticide level

FATS & OILS

Best: Whole, unrefined fats including raw grass-fed butter (if tolerated); ghee; tallow from grass-fed cows, bison, and lamb; lard from pasture-raised pigs; schmaltz from pasture-raised chickens and single-source organic extra-virgin olive oil; organic and sustainably farmed palm and coconut oils; organic cold-pressed sesame oil, nut oils, and avocado oil; fair-trade, organic cocoa butter
Better: Cultured butter made from organic pasteurized milk; conventionally produced extra-virgin olive oil; refined coconut oils and avocado oils
Good: Butter; light olive oil (not mixed with canola or other vegetable oils)
⊘ **Limit or Avoid:** Margarine; corn oil; soybean oil; canola oil; cottonseed oil; other vegetable oils; shortening and hydrogenated fats

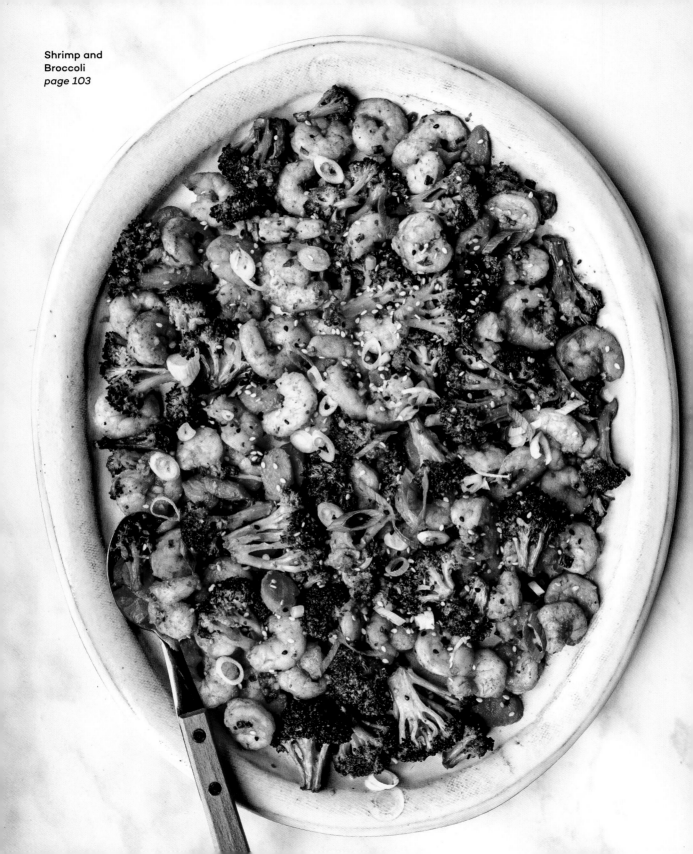

Shrimp and
Broccoli
page 103

Find Local Food and Source the Best Produce

Check out EatWild.com to search for local farms producing pasture-raised meats, dairy, and eggs in your area.

Check out Seafoodwatch.org for more about sustainable fish.

Check out local farmers' markets and community-supported agriculture (a.k.a. CSAs)—memberships or subscriptions providing you with a box of local, seasonal produce and more. Use LocalHarvest.org to find what's near you.

Use the Dirty Dozen and Clean 15 lists, which are updated yearly by the Environmental Working Group, at EWG.org.

When buying fresh produce, choose what's in season. To see what's in season locally to your area, checkout SeasonalFoodGuide.org.

Keep in mind that frozen produce is a great option. It's usually flash frozen at peak ripeness and freshness and is very convenient to ensure you have a diverse produce stash to cook from. Just read the labels before you buy to ensure there aren't additives.

Visit foodbymars.com/book-guide for more resources and recommendations.

Money-Saving Tips

Using the Paleo template doesn't mean blowing through a whole paycheck on your grocery bill. Over time, it should ideally save you money on groceries and health bills. Here are my best tips for making this a stress-free part of your health journey—one you can enjoy instead of sweating over dollars and cents!

Always have a grocery list and shopping plan.
First take inventory of your fridge, freezer, and pantry. Make a list of what you need. If you're trying a new recipe from this book or meal plan, see what you have already and shop for the rest.

Use fresh and frozen foods.
Price out fresh versus frozen and go with what's most convenient and affordable to you. Having frozen foods on hand is convenient, nutritious, and cost-effective. When shopping for fresh produce, try to stick with seasonal foods. They'll be more affordable, with less of a carbon footprint, and will also be more nutrient-dense. Try butternut squash, cabbage, collard greens, kale, rutabagas, sweet potatoes, or turnips.

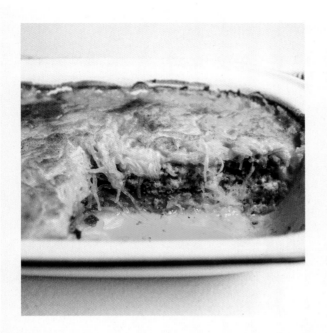

Food Deserts and Food Insecurity

Health is a basic right for everyone. If you have limited options, use the cost-saving tips provided here and look to community gardens, government-run programs (e.g., SNAP and WIC), local charities, and food banks (including mobile food banks like Meals on Wheels). Adding more whole foods into your diet is possible (no matter to what degree), and it will always help. If this is a cause you are interested in, donate or volunteer! Paying it forward in service is absolutely a healthy practice, too.

Shop organic only when necessary.
Shopping for organic produce is strongly encouraged to avoid consuming pesticides, antibiotics, and other toxins, but it's only needed for certain crops.

Make the cheaper "cuts" as your staples.
There are more affordable cuts of meat and types of seafood you can lean on while getting them from quality sources. For example, try chuck roast in the Instant Pot Beef Stew (page 72), pork butt/shoulder in Instant Pot Pernil (page 77), or even canned or frozen seafood (pages 143, 144, and 56).

Shop the sales and use the internet.
Search for local farms or look for discounts on shippable produce, animal products, and pantry items. When you find a good deal, buy in bulk and freeze the extra for later.

Know what to save on and what to splurge on.
Invest in kitchen tools you will use, such as an electric pressure cooker (e.g., Instant Pot) or cast-iron skillet. Quality pantry items and cooking staples, and even your own little herb garden, also pay off by elevating the flavors and nutrient density of your meals.

Start where you are, and have fun in the kitchen.
Small habits win the day, so don't bother racing to an invisible finish lane, stressing yourself out. As you try these practices, they'll fit into the larger ecosystem of your lifestyle and you will reap the benefits in both the short and long term.

#4 Anti-Inflammatory Whole Foods

Focusing solely on eliminations is a common pitfall of healing diets. Instead, concentrate on all the new vibrant foods you are adding to your diet! Cooking with healing, anti-inflammatory foods such as ginger, turmeric, and extra-virgin olive oil is a great way to use food as medicine. Also keep in mind that when it comes to many whole foods, one person's medicine can be another's poison. It's bio-individual! The beauty of this journey is experimenting with all sorts of new, delicious, nourishing ingredients.

You'll find these foods used throughout this book, sometimes as a seasoning or flavor addition and other times as a more "therapeutic" or medicinal dose! They're multifunctional.

Aloe Vera Juice

Aloe vera is packed with nutrients and contains many enzymes that are known to assist in the breakdown of sugars and fats (to keep digestion running smoothly). It can help decrease irritation in the stomach and intestines (to provide relief for IBS symptoms and other inflammatory disorders of the intestines). It can also assist in soothing inflammation in the upper GI tract. Drinking 100 percent whole leaf, unsweetened aloe vera juice can provide relief from heartburn and reflux, and also be taken 15 to 30 minutes before a meal as a preventative to such symptoms. Try an aloe vera drink or tonic on page 176 or 179.

Bone Broth

Bone broth is a rich source of bioavailable nutrients that support numerous aspects of a healthy body, including collagen, gelatin, and key gut-healing amino acids like glutamine and glycine. It also has some minerals (but most mineral content comes from vegetables). It supports your body's framework with amazing gelatin and collagen, and it soothes and repairs the gut lining.

Include broth as a regular staple in the diet as a cooking liquid, a drink or tonic, and in soups and stews. With any digestive disorders or illness, there's a benefit to using short- or long-cooked broths, but bio-individuality should always be applied. See page 40 and 42 for more details about broth types and uses.

Cardamom

This delightful spice has been used for thousands of years to help with digestion, often mixed with other medicinal spices such as ginger and cinnamon, to relieve discomfort, nausea, and vomiting. There's also research on its support of healing ulcers. And, cardamom may help to lower blood sugar. It also tastes delicious; you'll recognize the flavors from chai. Try it in the Rose-Cardamom Marshmallow Root Tea (page 170) or the No-Churn Blueberry Cardamom Nice Cream (page 157).

Cinnamon (Ceylon Cinnamon)

Cinnamon lowers blood sugar levels, slowing the breakdown of carbohydrates in your digestive tract (to get this medicinal effect regularly, you'll need ½ to 2 teaspoons of Ceylon cinnamon per day). This is key to regulating your energy and hormones, including those used for hunger/satiation. For a delicious way to add more cinnamon to your diet, make the Sautéed Cinnamon Apples with Yogurt (page 154).

Cloves

In some animal studies, clove extract and clove oil has been shown to increase the production of gastric mucus and help protect against stomach ulcers. Compounds in cloves may also help with blood sugar regulation, similarly to cinnamon. Enjoy cloves in your Gold Bone Broth Latte (page 169) or Rooibos Chai (page 177).

Coconut Oil

Cold-pressed extra-virgin coconut oil may have antimicrobial, antifungal, and antiviral effects through its lauric, capric, and caprylic acids. When you digest the lauric acid, the body forms monolaurin, which can kill harmful pathogens such as bacteria, viruses, and fungi.

Enzyme-Rich Fruits

Fruits such as papaya, pineapple, pears, apples, and more are rich in digestion supportive enzymes that assist in the breakdown of key nutrients. These make a great addition to sweet desserts and savory meals. Try some Chicken Pad Thai with Green Papaya Noodles (page 147) or Pineapple, Lime, and Mint Sorbet (page 156)!

Fennel Seeds

Fennel seeds can assist with bloating, gas, and GI cramping. Try the Green Minestrone Soup with Sausage (page 67) for a boost of fresh fennel *and* fennel seeds.

Fermented Foods

Fermented foods such as sauerkraut and yogurt are loaded with live active cultures, or probiotics. The tart or sour flavors help to stimulate digestive acids. As always, apply bio-individuality here especially, starting with low doses to see how you do with different types and in different amounts and frequencies. For example, try a forkful of the Fermented Coleslaw (page 184) with one meal a day and tweak from there. Test a few spoonfuls of Instant Pot Coconut Yogurt (page 187) as a topping on sautéed apples.

Ginger

Ginger can help increase gut motility. This is especially helpful for slow digestion or constipation. It can soothe gas pains in adults and babies, and is helpful for relieving nausea and often recommended to cancer patients undergoing chemo and radiation. Ginger is also known for its anti-inflammatory properties and in studies, has been shown in a combination with turmeric to be more effective than NSAIDs at reducing inflammation. Try the Creamy Ginger, Pear, and Butternut Squash Soup (page 64) or Bone Broth Ramen (page 68) for tasty ways to get more ginger in your diet.

Lavender

Lavender has been shown in studies to help ease stress and anxiety and promote more restful sleep. Because of the gut-brain connection, if you're able to rest your nerves and feelings of stress or anxiousness, you are supporting your gut health and digestive state. Lavender also is a bitter herb; bitters are helpful in stimulating digestive acids and bile production, and it can also ease stomach and intestinal cramps. Used in supplement, tincture-form, as a dried herb, or topically as an essential oil are the many ways to use this amazing herb for rest, relaxation, and supporting your gut-brain harmony. My recipe for Lavender Concentrate (page 179) is delicious in lemonade and tea.

Lemon Juice

In the Gut Refresh Meal Plan (page 196), I recommend starting your days off with warm or room temperature lemon water because of how amazing it is at stimulating digestion, elimination, and bile production, while supporting hydration. Using lemon juice in cooking, for drinking, and as a garnish are all great ways to get this digestion and liver supportive fruit into your diet regularly. Try the Lemon and Ginger Aloe Vera Tonic (page 176) and Lemony Greek Fisherman's Soup (page 59)

Marshmallow Root

This soothing herb can help digestive discomfort and flare-ups. It's commonly brewed as a tea (see page 170 for a delicious recipe for Rose-Cardamom Marshmallow Root Tea). It's a huge support during gut-healing protocols, as it helps with conditions all along the GI tract from the mouth, stomach, intestines, and bowels while also supporting the bladder, too!

Organ Meats

Organ meats, or offal, are a healing and strengthening food. The nutrient density outweighs that of the muscle meats we consume normally. Organ meats are more concentrated in vitamins, minerals, essential fatty acids, and essential amino acids. They're also a bio-available way to get these nutrients into the body for easy absorption. Try the delicious Mushroom Truffle Pâté (page 194), and don't stop trying to incorporate organ meats! You can sneak them into meatballs, hashes (page 94), or if needed, capsulated in supplements.

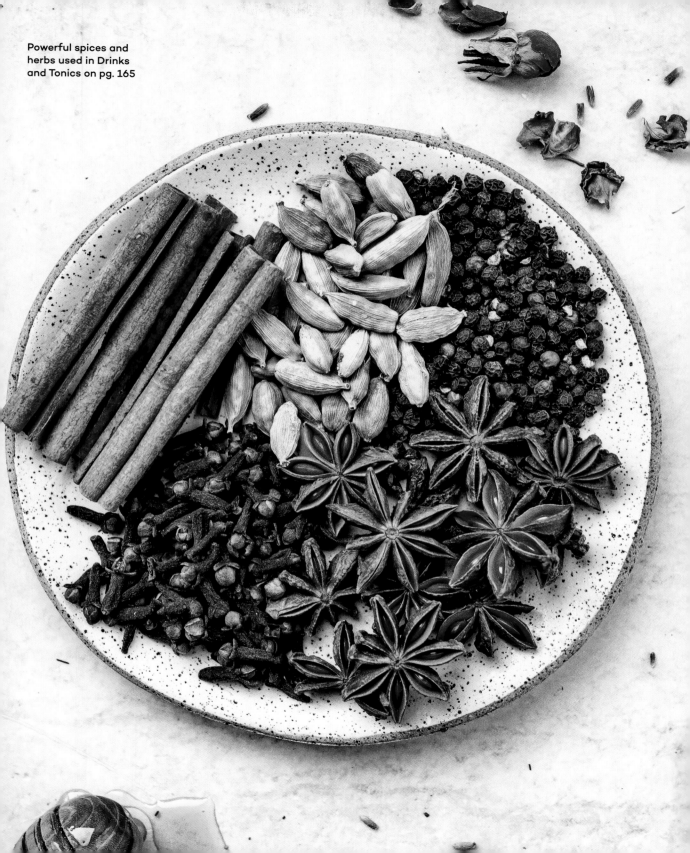

Powerful spices and herbs used in Drinks and Tonics on pg. 165

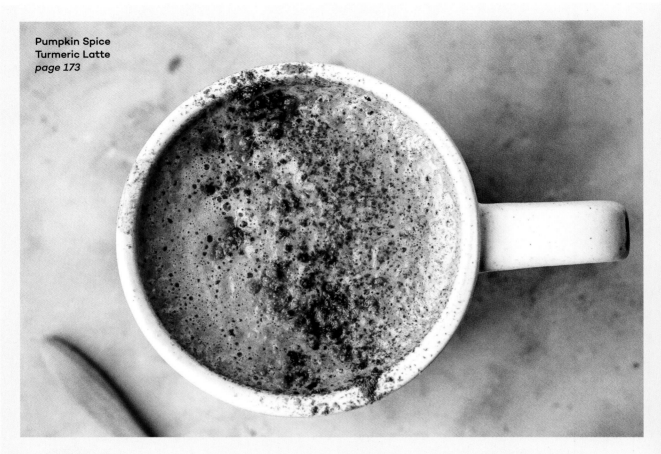

**Pumpkin Spice
Turmeric Latte**
page 173

Prebiotic-Rich Foods

Your beneficial gut bacteria rely on prebiotic fiber and resistant starches for food. Including these vegetables and fruits regularly and balanced with protein and fat helps to nourish your microbiome. If certain types like artichokes, plantains, or garlic cause any discomfort, just be mindful of the dose: Start low and slow, working your way up and listening to your body on how much you can handle, and how frequently. See page xx for more on adding prebiotics and probiotics into your diet.

Turmeric

Turmeric is a powerful anti-inflammatory and also helps stimulate bile production for the digestion and emulsification of fats. When combined with ginger, it's even been a more effective option at reducing inflammation than NSAIDs. The list of benefits goes on and on. When cooking with turmeric, be sure to combine it with a healthy fat such as coconut milk or ghee, for example, with a pinch of black pepper for optimal absorption. The piperine in pepper helps the body absorb the curcumin by up to 2,000%! This has been used for a long time in Ayurveda. Cozy up with a cup of Pumpkin Spice Turmeric Latte (page 173) or a Gold Bone Broth Latte (page 169). Keep it in your cooking spice cabinet, and you can even find it in supplement form to pop for a headache or take as a part of your daily routine if you and your health care professional agree!

#5 Prioritize Variety

Digestive issues and leaky gut are commonly tied to food sensitivities. Working with a practitioner on food sensitivity testing and protocols, eliminations, and challenging reintroductions may help you. During that work and afterward, you need to be careful not to lean too hard on the same foods repeatedly, or you may just become sensitive to those too!

We are creatures of habit, but we must be mindful that the poison is in the dose. Remember, once intestinal permeability or leaky gut is present or you're already noticing some food sensitivities, it's a slippery slope to having more. What you're eating a lot of may slip out through the intestinal lining and trigger your immune system to fight it as it would a foreign invader.

Another major reason to prioritize more variety of foods is because the diversity of your gut bacteria requires a diversity of foods, specifically from whole fruits and vegetables. By providing your microbiome with a variety of food, you'll promote having many species of healthy bacteria in the gut. You may supplement with probiotics for this but, as Dr. Datis Kharrazian has observed, one of the most effective ways to feed a diverse gut microbiome is by eating plentiful amounts of many kinds of vegetables and fruits for balance within the microbiome.

Ways to Try New Foods

There are so many ways to introduce new foods into your diet and vary the foods you eat. Try some of these strategies and you're sure to find new favorites and satisfy the pickiest of eaters.

→ Introduce things slowly through trial and error, and try foods that taste like familiar ones. For example, I often use rutabaga in place of white potatoes. Try using half rutabaga and half potatoes to start.

→ Season food with your favorite spices and add some sauce. My favorite chimichurri (page 191) pairs well with any protein or veggie you can throw at it!

→ Try a CSA (community-supported agriculture) subscription to get local, seasonal foods. Or look at seasonal lists for your part of the world and pick out some produce you haven't tried before!

→ Look for new varieties of your favorite produce. Love butternut squash? Try sunshine or buttercup squash for a bit of a change. Or seek out different colors of cabbage, cauliflower, and carrots with different phytonutrients.

→ Eat the rainbow. It's a fun visual way to make a beautiful plate. Try mixed, frozen vegetables or make your own mix. Use these in sautés and soups, or roast them in the oven. You won't get sick of the same vegetables repeatedly, and neither will your gut!

→ Prepare foods in a new way. For example, if you only ever roast veggies, try them in a sauté with new spices and herbs. Try steaming them. Puree them. "Rice" them. Turn them into veggie noodles.

→ Try a new animal protein. Have you tried bison/buffalo? How about elk? Venison? Duck or quail eggs?

→ Cook creatively! Try new recipes that expose you to new foods. And try new foods that inspire you to seek out new recipes.

Rotate Your Foods!

Many elimination diets, including some gut-healing therapeutic diets, don't exclude 100 percent of a whole food on the "avoid" list. Instead, there's an emphasis on the quantity of that particular food you are able to enjoy while healing. Again, the poison is in the dose. This can feel difficult to take on because we favor certain foods we like and tend to go all in on them. So, keep it simple . . . just keep switching it up and playing with quantities.

First, add a new variety of food. Swap out that almond milk in your coffee and use coconut milk instead! Or you can mix up your salad greens: One day it's arugula, and the next it's baby spinach. Add before you reduce or rotate; you want more variety, not less.

If you may be mildly sensitive to a food, or if you lean on it heavily and want to prevent developing a sensitivity to it, space the rotation out even more by three or four days. There's no hard-and-fast rule here. Try this and notice how you feel. Often a simple rotation system can clear up some symptoms and release attachment to certain foods—all while discovering new things you like even more!

Why You Need a Variety of Vegetables in Your Diet

A variety of vegetables in the diet helps to promote a variety of bacteria in the gut microbiome. Dr. Terry Wahls is a physician who reversed her multiple sclerosis through a very nutrient-dense Paleo template, going from a wheelchair back to her beloved bicycle. Her research showed that vegetables contain thirty-one micronutrients that our bodies require to heal, so the focus on quality, variety, and quantity of vegetables in the diet was a linchpin to her healing transformation.

#6 Sleep, Stress Management, and Moving Your Body

Sleep and stress are the most common blockers I see to true healing and good health. They seem to go hand-in-hand: If you're sleep deprived, it's a stressor on your body and mind. If you're stressed-out and riddled with anxiety and racing thoughts, you won't be able to achieve quality sleep. It can be a vicious cycle.

Getting Enough Quality Sleep

The circadian rhythm, or body clock, is a big part of how our bodies regulate. When it is thrown off, digestion, hormones, blood sugar, detoxification, and more are also thrown off. When you achieve deep sleep for around eight hours per night, your whole health is supported. Quality sleep ensures adequate growth hormone secretion from the pituitary to repair the tissues of the body, including the mucosal lining of the digestive system. During quality sleep, the digestive system can rest and repair. In addition, the function of many digestive enzymes requires appropriate circadian signaling. When imbalanced, the liver and pancreas, among other digestive organs, will fall behind.

When quality sleep is achieved, a rising level of prolactin during the night then leads to elevations of dopamine upon waking, providing us with a natural appetite control. However, if you lack quality sleep, normal hormonal function is thrown off, which can often drive us to poor food choices. Ghrelin levels (associated with the feeling of hunger) increase, and its companion hormone that brings the feeling of satiation (leptin) is suppressed.

Tips to Promote Quality Sleep

Go to bed early to sync closely with light and dark cycles for your circadian rhythm. Wake up early and at a similar time, consistently.

Get sun on your skin when you wake up. Open up those curtains—bonus if you can go right outside for a few minutes!

Get outside daily for a walk before work, and sit by a window, even on a cloudy day.

Wear blue-blocking glasses when using devices, and limit device use in the late evening and early morning hours.

Limit caffeine to one cup before noon only or experiment with giving it up.

Allow your digestion to rest and don't eat right before bed (especially with upper GI issues, such as reflux and heartburn), or it will compromise your sleep.

Form a consistent nighttime routine and practice good sleep hygiene. Keep your room quiet, dark, and cool (between 60 and 67 degrees).

Stress Management and Your Gut

Stress comes in many shapes and sizes. We all commonly experience psychological or emotional stress. Then there is the physiological stress that comes from the body doing its best to function optimally—against all the odds stacked against it, such as overwork, toxicity, and processed foods. Added to this is how we perceive stress based on our own life experiences, and possibly even those genetically or epigenetically programmed into us by our ancestors.

When the body is responding to a stressor or trigger, it's what is known as "the stress response," and we go into the sympathetic, or "fight or flight," nervous state. The body is perceiving danger. Whether it's an attacker or you're running late in traffic, the body isn't distinguishing; it's reacting to save your life in either scenario. In this state, the body has to de-prioritize everything else it's doing, including digestion.

Our bodies are so beautifully designed to save our lives, but this response wasn't intended to be triggered every single day, multiple times a day. And in our stressful modern-day lives of traffic, deadlines, arguments, alarming news headlines, bills, being sedentary workaholics, processed foods, too much sugar, too much caffeine, chronic antibiotic use . . . we are beating our body (especially our adrenals) up constantly, and it's causing a cascading effect on our health.

Chronic stress affects digestion, blood sugar regulation, fatty acid sufficiency, inflammation, minerals, metabolism and weight, hormone balance, and general mental health. If you're a person who says things like "I'm not that stressed" or "Well, it could be much worse," I invite you to check in on that. Many of us have developed quite a high threshold for stress and can be out of tune with our relationship to it and how it's affecting us physically. And emerging research by Dr. David Rakel, M.D., via the Institute for Functional Medicine suggests stress may also be a causal factor in gut dysbiosis (bacterial imbalances).

We can't just run away from all our problems or escape stress. It's a part of our daily lives. But we can and must balance it out with stress management. Employing daily techniques such as mindfulness (page 24), meditation, self-care, and gratitude journaling can help us cope with our stress.

Another great way to manage stress and care for your body is to move it! This can mean a rigorous workout or a simple foundation of daily movement. How about dancing in the morning with the sun hitting your skin? Grounding your feet in the backyard without shoes while you enjoy your morning coffee or tea? Yoga or stretching in the morning or last thing before bed? Going for a 30-minute walk in your neighborhood after lunch to give your brain a reset with some fresh air and get circulation going?

And if you feel like you don't have enough time in the day to be active, keep in mind that sitting for long periods of time, staring at screens, and contorting our bodies with poor posture are not ideal for digestion. Staying stagnant in the body will cause a stagnant or sluggish digestive system, add to stress in the body, and even make sleep more restless. Try adding movement to your day when you can and see how it helps in your stress management, digestion, and sleep. Every little bit helps!

4, 7, 8 Breathing Technique

This technique developed by Dr. Andrew Weil is a powerful breathing exercise to activate the relaxation response in the body. Try four rounds per day or whenever you're feeling anxious or stressed out.

→ Inhale through the nose for four counts.
→ Hold for seven counts.
→ Exhale through the mouth for eight counts.

Exercising Your Vagus Nerve to Activate the Parasympathetic Nervous System

The vagus nerve, which runs from your gut to your brain, is a linchpin for your gut health and overall health. By activating this nerve, you enter the parasympathetic state. This helps you to manage stress, rest and digest, and support your immunity. As with any body part, the more you use it, the stronger it will be!

Here are ways to exercise or activate the vagus nerve:

→ Meditation (even for a few minutes per day)

→ Mindfulness and mindful eating

→ Slow, rhythmic, diaphragmatic breathing (belly/diaphragm breathing vs. in your chest/lungs alone)

→ Humming and singing loudly (in the shower, as you drive, or go about chores . . . go for it!)

→ Gargling water for at least thirty seconds per day

→ Using essential oils formulated for vagus nerve

→ An ice pack to the cheeks or under the ear, a cold shower, or cold water on the face

#7 Incorporating Broths and Prebiotic- and Probiotic-Rich Foods

Broth is a powerful tool for healing and sealing the gut lining. Use it for sipping, as a cooking liquid, in soups, and even in smoothies! Bone broths are widely available, both frozen and shelf-stable—and luckily, making your own broths at home is also really simple. Homemade is affordable, reliable, and the best way to eat nose to tail.

Creating a broth-making routine need not be hard, expensive, or time-consuming. It can be a "set it and forget it" type of routine you do as frequently as you'd like, and it will provide you with crucial nutrients you need for gut healing.

Broth Making

All you need are bones, filtered water, something acidic such as apple cider vinegar or lemon juice, and any herbs or vegetables you'd like to throw in there! For long-cooked bone broths, I recommend avoiding cruciferous/bitter vegetables or sweet vegetables, as they might overflavor the broth with bitterness or sweetness. Check out my recipes on page 182 (basic broth) and page 183 (bone broth).

For sourcing bones, it's easiest to save them from the meat you cook and eat regularly. You can also ask your butcher for leftover bones. Simply cook those in the oven before using. Buying chicken feet to freeze and save as an add-in is also a great idea and produces a very rich broth.

To make broth, a simple Dutch oven or a large soup pot is all you need. Simmer all the ingredients over low heat for several hours. This is the traditional way our ancestors went about it. I love using a slow cooker simply because it's electric and can be placed out of the way for a long period of time. Mine is also large and can make a lot of broth. You may also use an electric pressure cooker (Instant Pot).

Save the fat! If a layer of fat rises to the top of your basic broth or bone broth after being cooled, spoon off that top fat layer and save it in a separate jar to use as cooking fat. Try using it in mashed cauliflower (page 125) or in a skillet meal (page 84).

To store the broth, use freezer-safe jars. I recommend mason jars in various sizes; you may want smaller ones some weeks and larger ones other weeks. I also use silicone ice cube trays to freeze broth and then transfer them to a freezer bag or container for use in cooking liquid or heating up a quick mug for sipping!

Homemade Broth Made Easy

One and done: Make a whole chicken on a regular basis (every Sunday or every other week). Toss the carcass right in the slow cooker or pot to make the broth. See how long broth normally lasts you and you can plan your chicken meal around that!

Stockpile: Store all leftover bones from your meals in a freezer bag or freezer-safe container. Once a freezer bag is full, it's time to make broth!

Vary the flavors: Try seasonal herbs or vegetables with your broths. In the winter, maybe you're craving more red meat broths. In the warmer months, maybe more poultry or fish is your jam! Have fun—make this your own, and adjust it to your own tastes.

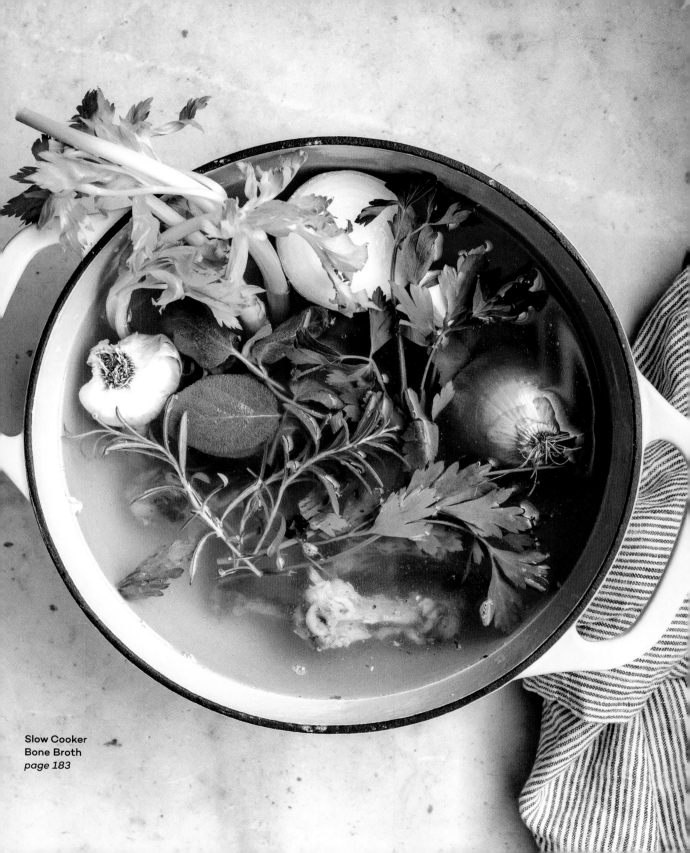

Slow Cooker
Bone Broth
page 183

Broth Nutrition and Benefits

Broth is a staple in many healing diets. It's prevalent in the Paleo diet as it's a traditional food, and it's used in the Autoimmune Protocol (AIP) diet as a part of healing the gut while removing inflammatory triggers and challenging reintroductions.

Bone broth (page 183) is long-cooked (12 to 48 hours) with just bones as the base. The top four amino acids found in bone broth are glycine, glutamine, proline, and alanine. All amino acid levels are about three times higher in long-cooked broth than in short-cooked broth, but they are still present in short-cooked broths.

Basic broth (page 182) is short-cooked (two to six hours) often with both bones and meat. This is the broth you'd usually make as a byproduct of homemade chicken soup. If a person is suffering with histamine intolerance, or severe gut distress, and doesn't seem to respond well to bone broth, try a short-cooked broth instead, as it may be easier to digest and tolerate for some.

Stocks are similar to bone broths, using bones as the base, but not cooked as long, and can also be used in the recipes. If you're keen on learning more about the healing power of broths, see my resources section on page 201.

Prebiotics and Probiotics

Prebiotic foods such as asparagus, Jerusalem artichoke, and green plantains are food for your gut bacteria. Including a variety of vegetables in your diet will provide your gut with the food it needs for diversity. Probiotics add to your gut bacteria. Including fermented foods in your routine will add more diversity to the gut. You want a healthy mix of both.

Go low and slow with these. Start with a forkful of fermented vegetables such as sauerkraut, kimchi, or Fermented Coleslaw (page 184) at a meal. Add a dollop of Instant Pot Coconut Yogurt (page 187) on some sautéed apples (page 154). Move from there in quantity and frequency as you see fit. Everyone will react differently and may need different amounts at different times. Make your own or look for brands with minimal ingredients. See what feels good.

#8 Avoid "Junk" Foods and Allergens

By following a Paleo and/or AIP template, you're already kicking out processed foods, refined sugars, and other "junk" that can impede gut health. The easiest way to abstain from these foods is to crowd your plate with vibrant, nutrient-dense foods. Use more natural, low-glycemic sweeteners and whole fruit. Rely on fewer processed pantry items with minimal ingredients and be sure they are Paleo-friendly. This can still provide you with an 80/20 diet (80 percent healthful changes and 20 percent indulgences), so you're able to enjoy conveniences and favorite foods, but without eating harmful additives.

Hyperpalatable and processed foods tend to suppress or overwrite hunger and satiation cues in the body. This means you won't feel full and you'll keep eating! Think about how you might eat a whole bag of chips, but can only eat one apple! After not having sugary, hyperpalatable foods in your diet, your hunger and satiation hormones (ghrelin and leptin) will normalize and your digestion will also improve.

I'm a huge advocate for having your Paleo cake and eating it too. If you love to bake some Paleo-friendly cookies on a Sunday after meal prep and you can enjoy them in moderation without them taking hold of you or your health, that's awesome! If your digestion is severely impaired and you simply can't handle it, then it's just not the time for it, but maybe one day it can be.

Indulging in a dessert will always best serve your body and soul when it's done mindfully and happily. It's about the action and purpose behind the snack or dessert. If you're in a stressed-out, anxious, sympathetic state, that snack is throwing your blood sugar and detox pathways off. You may have times when treats are off the table for you because they are being used to cope or escape stress and emotions. Know thyself and pull back.

Progress over Perfection

When you want to approach treats, do so mindfully using the best ingredients possible. That's all. No hard and fast rules here. It may take some "self-parenting" as I like to call it! Make the right decision for your healing body in the moment, own it, and move on. There's nothing wrong with finding a balance and enjoying life on your terms.

Keep in mind that this doesn't have to be all or nothing, if you don't want that. It simply has to be what you need at the present time. Honor it, don't judge, and move on so it can stop being an obstacle and a fight. Stop giving it brain power, and you give it less power altogether.

A word on Paleo-friendly treats: Even Paleo baked goods can sometimes be loaded with almond flour, coconut flour, and eggs—things that, in excess, might cause sluggish digestion. When you're working on healing your gut, perhaps one serving will be totally fine or perhaps not. Maybe it's a gateway to eating five servings! Use your best judgment. Abstain if you have to for your health.

Ways to Curb Sugar Cravings

Brush your teeth and scrape your tongue after consuming dessert or sweets.

Crowd it out with whole foods: Enjoy sweet vegetables and whole fruit as snacks. Use a bit of coconut oil and cinnamon to help stabilize blood sugar, or try almond butter if consuming nuts!

Check your protein and fat intake. Make sure you're getting enough because both will help curb sugar cravings and keep you satiated for longer between meals.

Stay hydrated between meals. Sometimes you might think you're hungry when it's actually dehydration.

Use self-care to soothe and comfort yourself. If you find you're "snacky" due to stress or boredom, identify what that feeling of snacking affords you. Perhaps it's just comfort or a way to pass the time.

Start savory! Have a savory, protein-rich breakfast that's low in starchy carbs and has no added sugars. (Watch your coffee/tea add-ins!) Starting your day this way avoids spiking your blood sugar, so there's no crash or sugar cravings the rest of the day.

Apply the 80/20 or 90/10 rule by prioritizing savory breakfasts (such as the Meat Hash with Kale and Cabbage on page 94) five to six days out of the week. This will keep you energized and focused most days, and your body can handle the occasional treat.

Practice mindful eating (page 24).

Get moving! The sugar in your body is meant to be a quick-burning energy source. Take a brisk walk, jog, go run your errands, dance, lift weights . . . whatever you like.

Practice daily gratitude. The mind-body connection is powerful. Taking just a few minutes to think about three things you're grateful for—even better to write them down! This practice changes your thought patterns and helps manage stress.

Breathe. Try the 4, 7, 8 breathing technique (page 39) once a day or at least when you're feeling anxious and stressed or battling a sweet tooth.

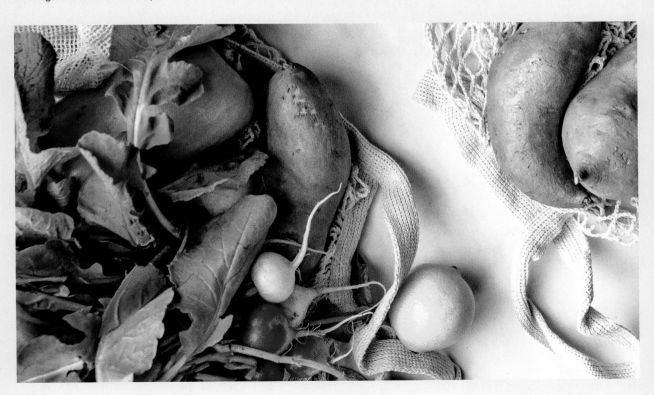

#9 Staying Well-Hydrated

It seems like the simplest thing to drink water, and yet dehydration is so commonplace. Why? The stories I normally hear from people struggling to stay hydrated are that they are "too busy and lose track of time," "don't have time to pee" (yes, that's real), and "water is boring!" This one practice done consistently can improve your health across the board. It will help you get better sleep, have more energy, experience smoother digestion and elimination, and more. Here's why:

→ Water helps transport nutrients all around your body.
→ Water improves oxygen delivery to cells and enables cellular hydration.
→ Water regulates body temperature.
→ Water helps cushion your joints and bones, while absorbing shock.
→ Water removes waste and flushes toxins.

Keep in mind that your body needs electrolytes. No, not from a colorful sports drink! Naturally occurring electrolytes help you hold on to enough water for use. Coconut water is packed with electrolytes from all the minerals like magnesium, sodium, and potassium. You can also simply add a pinch of mineral-rich, high-quality sea salt in your water for electrolytes, and a squeeze of lemon or lime juice would be a bonus for added vitamin C.

Ways to Be Sure You Stay Hydrated

How much water is enough? A general rule of thumb to follow is half your body weight in ounces, plus an additional 1½ cups (355 ml) for each caffeinated beverage or diuretic you consume. For example, if you weigh 150 pounds, you'd aim for 75 ounces of water per day (or about nine to ten cups). If you drink one coffee per day, you will chase it with an additional 1½ cups (355 ml) of water because the coffee dehydrates you and you must replace it.

If your hydration amount seems far off from what you normally drink in a day, best to work up to it. Once you've calculated it, go and invest in a nice glass water bottle and know how often per day you must refill it to hit your hydration amount! This will make it much easier to eyeball and keep track.

For digestion's sake, aim to take in most of your water between meals. Only sip the water you need during meals as opposed to gulping or chugging it. Room temperature or even slightly warm water is best for digestion.

If you're not keen on drinking water because of taste (or lack thereof), you can spruce it up by making a "spa water" with pieces of fruit. I love good old-fashioned lemon water, but try orange, lime, or strawberry. Pouring in some ginger tea or juice is a great way to support your gut motility and digestion, too!

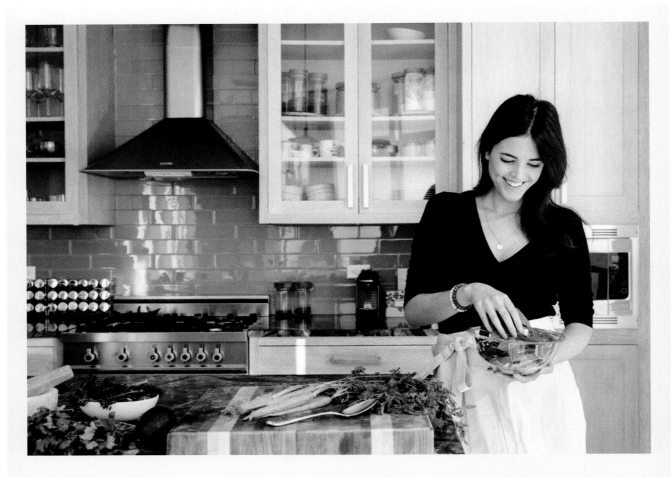

Filtering Your Water

Unfortunately, regardless of where your tap water is sourced, most water is exposed to pollutants, toxins, pharmaceuticals, and other contaminants. Many popular filters in the marketplace aren't strong or effective enough in filtering these very harmful toxins out of water, and it's vital to have clean water as you stay hydrated all day.

Do your research to ensure your water filter is kicking out as many toxins as possible, including arsenic, BPA, chlorine, chromium 6, fluoride, glyphosate (Roundup), lead, microplastics, pesticides, PFAs/PFOAs, radiation, and so on. You should be able to see a full report on any brand website (and if you can't, ditch it!). Visit foodbymars.com/book-guide for my recommended brands.

Signs of Dehydration

→ Fatigue
→ Anxiety
→ Irritability
→ Depression
→ Cravings
→ Cramps

→ Headaches
→ Heartburn
→ Joint pain
→ Back pain

→ Migraines
→ Fibromyalgia
→ Constipation
→ Colitis

#10 Preparing Food for Easy Digestion

Properly preparing food optimizes it for digestion and nutrient absorption. Some foods may require a little extra lovin', as I like to say, especially ones containing lectins. Most are excluded on the Paleo template (such as grains and legumes, which should be soaked/sprouted, and even pressure-cooked). If you add those back to your diet, just remember that! They may sit a whole lot better in your body when prepared properly and not rushed.

Soaking Nuts and Seeds

Nuts and seeds can benefit from being soaked. When soaked or sprouted, they're often called "activated" nuts and seeds. The process makes them much easier to digest while reducing phytic acid. Limit nuts and seeds to 1 ounce (28 g) or a palmful per day.

1. Place 4 cups (1 kg) of raw, shelled nuts into a large mixing bowl. (Weight will vary.)

2. Cover with water and stir in 1 tablespoon (17 g) of Celtic sea salt.

3. Soak for several hours (see table).

4. Drain and eat.

To store them in bulk, first drain the soaked nuts or seeds. Place in a dehydrator for 12 to 24 hours. Alternatively, spread the nuts on a large baking sheet lined with unbleached parchment paper and dehydrate them in a warm oven (under 150°F [66°C]) for 12 to 24 hours.

TYPE	SOAKING TIME
Almond	8–12 hours
Brazil nut	(do not soak)
Cashew	2 hours
Flax seed	8 hours
Hemp seed	(do not soak)
Macadamia	(do not soak)
Pecan	4–6 hours
Pepita (Pumpkin seed)	8 hours
Pistachio	(do not soak)
Sesame seed	8 hours
Sunflower seed	2 hours
Walnut	4 hours

Preparing Vegetables

There are optimal ways to prepare vegetables for easier digestion. For example, steaming broccoli or cauliflower instead of eating them raw can eliminate symptoms of gas or cramping they may otherwise cause. Try roasted or sautéed vegetables. I've found that some cruciferous vegetables such as broccoli, when roasted too long, bother me and cause stomach pain. When steamed and drizzled with extra-virgin olive oil and lemon juice, I could eat cups and cups of it! You might find you enjoy cooked vegetables over raw salad depending on the day, season, or stage of healing you're in.

**Moussaka
(Greek Eggplant
Casserole)
page 109**

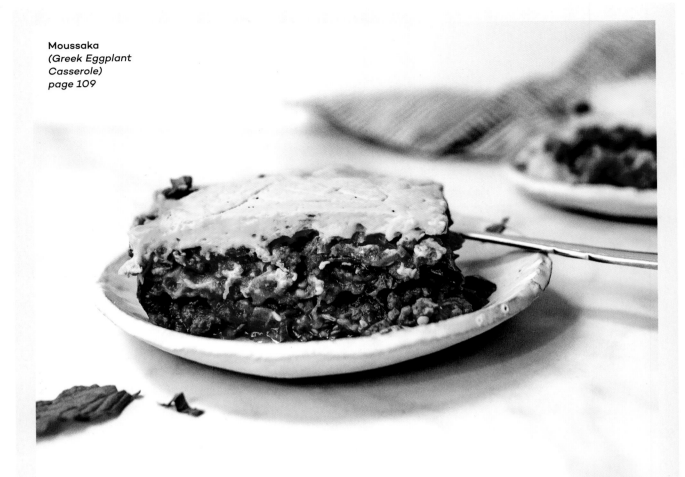

Cooking vegetables with broth as the cooking liquid, in a sauté, or in a soup is also helpful for digestion. (I've got plenty of veggie soups coming your way!) Combining this with healthy fats and healthy cooking oils is also helpful in absorption. If fresh aromatics such as onion and garlic bother you, try garlic and onion powders instead with other spices or seasonings.

Mindful eating (page 24) is also easier if you prepare food in smaller pieces by mashing it or cutting it up. Hello, cauliflower rice! Or puree it in soups to help you slow down and savor your food more effectively with little effort. Most important, don't fear food. Play with it! Listen to your body. Choose food that feeds you and heals you, while adding a few simple practices to your lifestyle. Above all else, *see what feels best for you*. Now, let's get into the kitchen and have some fun with the following recipes and two-week meal plan!

HOW TO USE THIS BOOK

As you've read, your gut healing journey is not just about what you eat. It's about how you eat, too. Use what you've just read to arm yourself with lifestyle tips and practices (with data) to try. And next, you'll get to use delicious recipes to integrate into your life, all while considering your bio-individuality.

My advice is to approach trying these new habits and recipes with curiosity to get more in tune with your body. You are building your personal lifestyle. Journal changes, results, symptoms, and other notes on your journey for this as well! You can visit foodbymars.com/book-guide for printable downloads like a food and mood journal and my most up-to-date product and resource recommendations. Practice progress over perfection. When trying anything new, I always recommend starting with one, two, maybe even three things at a time (for a week or two). Changes need time, and you want to be sure you've given it a fair shot and not bitten off more than you can chew.

If you're new to Paleo, I highly recommend starting with the Paleo template and sticking to that for at least one month consistently. The Autoimmune Protocol can be very beneficial for deeper healing and especially for those with autoimmune diseases, but only when practiced properly. So, if after trying Paleo (which should already support your gut health and various symptoms), you'd like to explore more interventions for improved symptom management, working up to AIP is the best way to set yourself up for success. Use the tips in this book, have a strong support system, and be sure you are up to the task to see the eliminations and the reintroductions through. The AIP diet can be challenging and isn't right for everyone all the time. Get support from a practitioner when you need it and above all, listen to your body and have fun. Enjoy!

Working with Your Doctor/Practitioner

The information in this book is meant for educational purposes only. Always check with your health care provider or medical practitioner when making changes. There may be underlying infections, overgrowths, or even parasites present when symptoms persist. Working with a functional/integrative doctor, naturopathic doctor, or other types of holistic practitioners will help you identify this through advanced testing.

You can search in your area or look for remotely operating doctors and practitioners if there are none available locally to you. These doctors and practitioners are trained to dig deeper, always looking for the root causes of your symptoms to address the foundations of your health. They may use different types of tests, medicine, and supplements, and recommend diet and lifestyle changes to assist in treatment. Medications also alter the gut microbiome, such as the birth control pill or proton-pump inhibitors (PPIs), and with a doctor's supervision, you may explore weaning off these medications if you will instead manage through diet and lifestyle.

Combining expert support with using everyday practices like the ones shared in this book is a powerful way to manage your gut health thoroughly and have all bases covered.

Recipe Icons

There is no separate breakfasts chapter in this book because one of the major shifts you'll make is to move away from sweet bowls, pancakes, and waffles. This change will automatically improve your digestion and blood sugar regulation. That said, I've got you covered with great ways to start your day! Just look for this icon throughout the book.

These meals are easiest to make on the fly, on a weeknight, or really any time at all!

Whether it's a roasted sheet pan of protein and veggies or a flavorful skillet, these meals require less dishwashing than the rest!

The recipe is AIP-friendly for the elimination phase of the Autoimmune Protocol as is. Most recipes have details about how to make it elimination-phase friendly. For the rare few that can't be adapted, you can always come back to them once you've reintroduced the ingredients to your diet.

Kitchen Tips and Tricks

Batch cooking is a great way to prepare full meals in advance to either freeze or store in the refrigerator. This is especially helpful for shift workers or people who travel a lot and can't schedule time to cook every day. It's also a good option for large families who always need meals ready to go.

"Cook once, eat twice" is more of a stockpiling style of preparing meals. If you're cooking for two people, cook for four and store the leftovers for an upcoming meal. Each time you do this, you're adding meals and maximizing your time spent in the kitchen. This works well for those who don't like leftovers or who don't have a ton of room in their kitchen storage for batch cooking.

"Half and half" is how I cook. On a Sunday I prepare some "base" meal options—such as ground meat or anything that takes longer than 45 minutes to cook. Then, throughout the week I have plenty of easy "accessories" to have a delicious ready-to-go meal in minutes.

Store and freeze vegetables in jars or freezer bags to roast, sauté, or steam later.

Make extra servings of soup. Fill a mason jar three-quarters of the way full, freeze, and then defrost for a quick meal.

Mince fresh garlic in bulk and freeze it on a flat surface. Then store in a freezer bag or jars to have on hand.

Freeze bone broths, fresh herbs in coconut or olive oil, and homemade sauces such as pesto or chimichurri in silicon ice cube trays. Then store in a jar or freezer bag once solid for easy access when cooking.

Store-Bought Ready-Made Snacks

If you're eating balanced meals throughout the day, your need to snack will likely be rare, but if you're caught traveling or find yourself hungry, you need to eat something! These ideas are super helpful to have on hand or in your purse.

→ Canned or pouched fish (e.g., tuna, sardines, or salmon)
→ Cassava chips
→ Unsweetened coconut flakes
→ Dried fruit with no sweeteners added (in moderation) such as dates, prunes, or pineapple
→ Dehydrated vegetables
→ Fresh fruit
→ Hard-boiled eggs
→ Olives
→ Raw or roasted nuts with no additives (omit for AIP)
→ Nut or seed butter pouches with no sweeteners or processed oils added (omit for AIP)
→ Raw vegetables (e.g., carrots and celery)
→ Plantain chips
→ Seaweed snacks
→ Seeds
→ Smoked fish (e.g., wild smoked salmon)
→ Sweet potato chips

Clutch Paleo Swaps

While Paleo products can be great, I always recommend leading with whole food replacements first. It will likely also save you money. The best swap is one that's minimally processed and as close to nature as possible!

Traditional Pasta → vegetable noodles or zoodles, spaghetti squash, rutabaga, etc.
Check out the Pesto Primavera Veggie Noodles with Shrimp (page 115), Chicken Zoodle Soup (page 60), or Chicken Pad Thai with Green Papaya Noodles (page 147).

Lasagna Noodles → thinly sliced vegetables such as butternut squash, eggplant, zucchini, plantains, or packed spaghetti squash
Check out the Pastelón (page 106), Spaghetti Squash Pastitsio (page 108), or Moussaka (page 109).

Rice → vegetable rice made from cauliflower, plantains, sweet potato, and broccoli.
Try the Veggie Confetti Rice (page 133).

Cheese → using nutritional yeast and lemon juice replicates a cheesy flavor
Try my "cheese" sauce using steamed cauliflower, coconut cream, and nutritional yeast (page 188)

Bread/wraps → plantains, sweet potato slices, collard greens, lettuce, cabbage, and just about any vegetable you can wrap food into!
Try my Greek Stuffed Cabbage Rolls in Lemony Sauce (page 112) and Mango Chicken Jibaritos (page 105).

Yogurt/sour cream → Instant Pot Coconut Yogurt (page 187) or other nondairy yogurt (e.g., almond/cashew without additives or sugar)

Butter → ghee, lard, tallow, palm shortening, solid coconut oil

Chips/crackers → plantain chips, cassava chips, seaweed snacks, sweet potato chips (all cooked in a healthy oil such as olive, palm, or coconut), nut/seed flour crackers, pork rinds

Croutons → any of the "chips/crackers" alternatives crushed on top of your salad, chopped nuts, or seeds

Fast café drinks → bone broth (get creative with your own flavorings), brewed at home fair-trade organic coffees and teas with full-fat coconut milk and raw honey or maple syrup instead of half-and-half or sugar

I have lovely drinks and tonics (pages 166 to 179) that your gut will love way more than their sugar-laden counterparts.

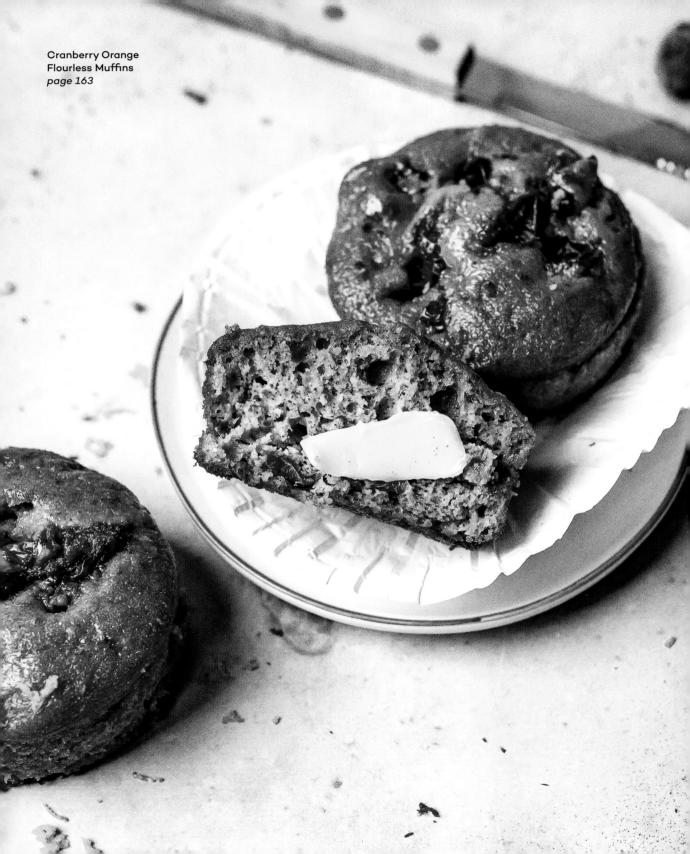

**Cranberry Orange
Flourless Muffins**
page 163

Lifesaving Kitchen Essentials

These will save you time and effort in the kitchen, making cooking much smoother so you can get back to other things!

→ Electric pressure cooker (Instant Pot)
→ Slow cooker (Crock Pot)
→ High-speed blender
→ Spiralizer
→ Cast-iron skillet
→ Stainless steel cookware (skillets, pots, pans)
→ Food processor
→ Dutch oven or stockpot
→ Casserole or baking dishes (glass, ceramic, or enamel)
→ Measuring cups and spoons
→ Silicon muffin trays and ice trays
→ Large slotted spoon
→ Vegetable peeler
→ Zester or microplane
→ Sieve or strainer
→ Wooden spoons
→ Mandoline slicer
→ Spice grinder/coffee grinder
→ Steam basket
→ Saucepan
→ Kitchen shears
→ Sharp knives
→ Unbleached parchment paper
→ Cutting board

Visit foodbymars.com/book-guide for more resources, reintroduction tips and a free journal download, money-saving tips, and the most up-to-date recommended products to guide you.

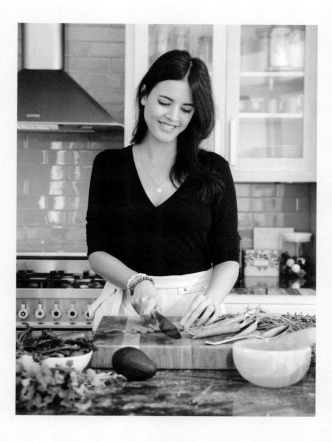

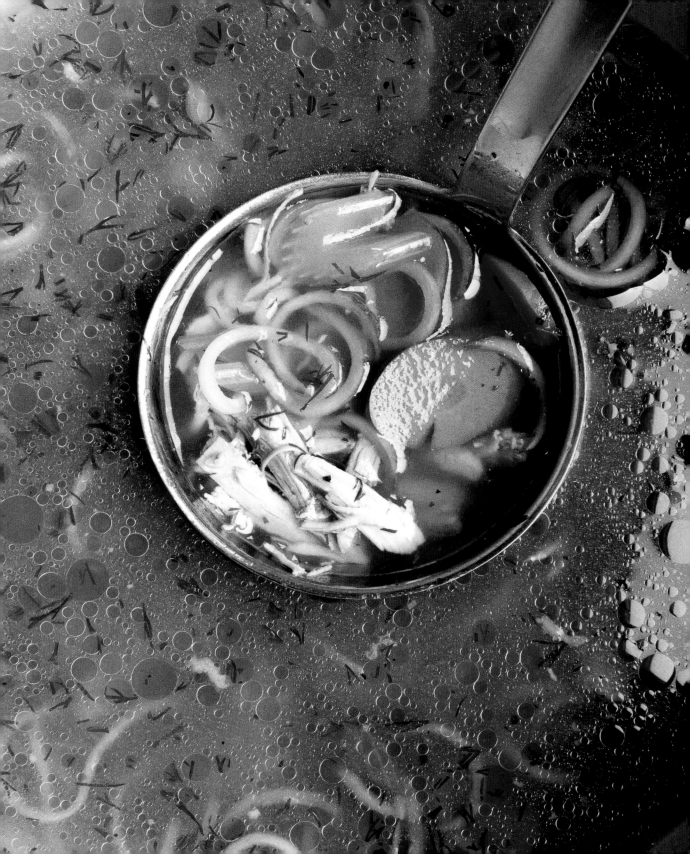

3

SOUPS & STEWS

Coming home to a warming bowl of soup or stew heals my gut just thinking about it! Made with rich broths and tons of vegetables, herbs, and seasonings, there's something here for everyone to enjoy. Some are easy to whip up on a weeknight, and others are more of a weekend project to prepare you for the week or devour on a chilly day spent at home. These soups make a great meal any time of day (even breakfast!), and they will nourish you from the inside out. I'm also sharing some time-saving electric pressure cooker recipes that are perfect for meal prepping.

Green Coconut Curry Shrimp Soup 56
Lemony Greek Fisherman's Soup *(Psarosoupa)* 59
Chicken Zoodle Soup 60
Italian Wedding Soup 63
Creamy Ginger, Pear, and Butternut Squash Soup 64
Green Minestrone Soup with Sausage 67
Bone Broth Ramen 68
Mushroom and Cauliflower Rice Soup with Chicken 71
Instant Pot Beef Stew 72
Instant Pot Shredded Chicken 74
Instant Pot Lamb Shanks 75
Instant Pot Pernil *(Garlic Pulled Pork)* 77

Green Coconut Curry Shrimp Soup

This cozy, rich soup is quick enough to make for a weeknight meal, but it tastes like it took much longer! The spices and creamy coconut will warm your belly, and the ginger and curry have anti-inflammatory properties. This will definitely beat your favorite takeout because you made it yourself with trusted ingredients.

PREP TIME 10 minutes
COOK TIME 15 minutes
TOTAL TIME 25 minutes
YIELD 4 servings

AIP-FRIENDLY GREEN CURRY PASTE
(Yield: about 16 ounces, or 455 g)

6 scallions, sliced

2 stalks lemongrass, chopped

2 tablespoons (12 g) minced ginger or 2½ teaspoons (4.5 g) powder

2 tablespoons (12 g) minced turmeric or 2½ teaspoons (5.5 g) powder

4 cloves garlic, minced

⅔ cup (10 g) chopped cilantro

Zest and juice of 1 lime

1 tablespoon (15 ml) maple syrup or raw honey

½ teaspoon sea salt

3 tablespoons (42 g) coconut or avocado oil, plus more if needed

SOUP
4 medium zucchinis or 4 cups (480 g) prepared zoodles

7 scallions

1 lime

4 small sweet peppers or 2 bell peppers, mixed colors (omit for AIP)

3 tablespoons (45 ml) extra-virgin olive oil, divided

1 knob (3 inches, or 7.5 cm) of ginger, peeled and thinly sliced

3–4 ounces (85–115 g) green curry paste (store-bought organic or an AIP version)

2 cans (13.5 ounces, or 383 g) unsweetened full-fat coconut milk, divided

¼ teaspoon sea salt

1½ pounds (680 g) large shrimp, peeled and deveined

2 cups (130 g) snap peas (omit for AIP)

¼ cup (4 g) chopped cilantro, plus more for garnish

To make the paste: Add all of the ingredients except the coconut oil to a food processor or blender. Pulse until well chopped. Add the coconut oil 1 tablespoon (14 g) at a time, pulsing until a paste forms. Set aside.

To make the soup: Spiralize the zucchinis, and add them to your serving bowls, and set aside. Chop the white and green parts of the scallions; slice and reserve the dark tops for garnish. Zest the lime and cut the lime into slices for garnish. Slice the peppers into rings or slices.

Over medium heat, add 2 tablespoons (30 ml) of oil to a medium saucepan with a lid. Add the scallions, zest, peppers, and ginger. Cook for 8 minutes, stirring often, until the veggies are golden. Add the curry paste to taste and stir for 2 to 3 minutes. Add 1½ cans of coconut milk. Stir, taste, and adjust the coconut milk or paste if needed. Season with salt. Reduce the heat to a low simmer. Cook for 6 minutes, stirring occasionally.

Add the shrimp, peas, and cilantro. Cover and cook for 2 to 3 minutes, until the shrimp is bright pink. Ladle your curry over the zoodles and garnish with dark scallion tops, lime slices, and cilantro.

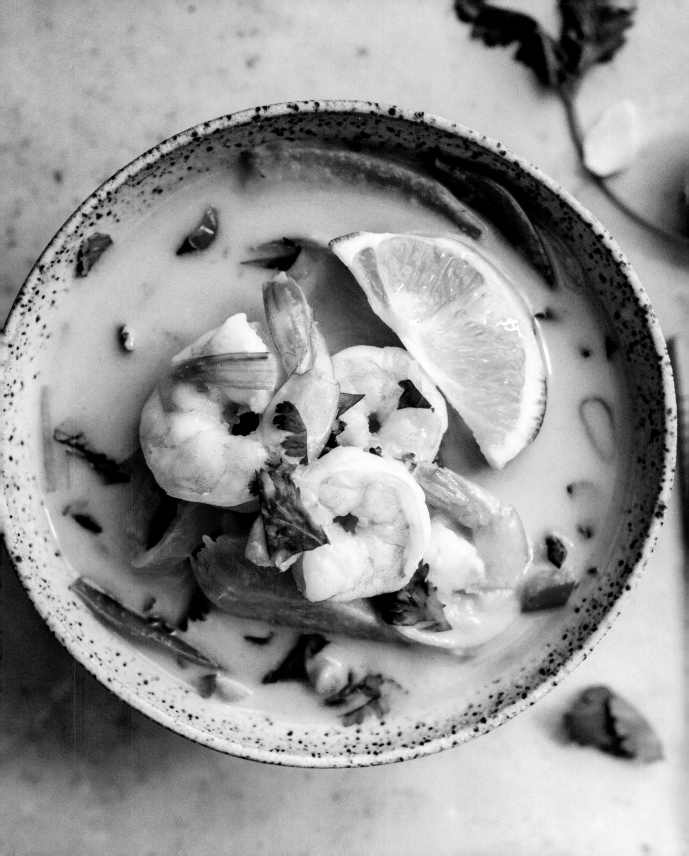

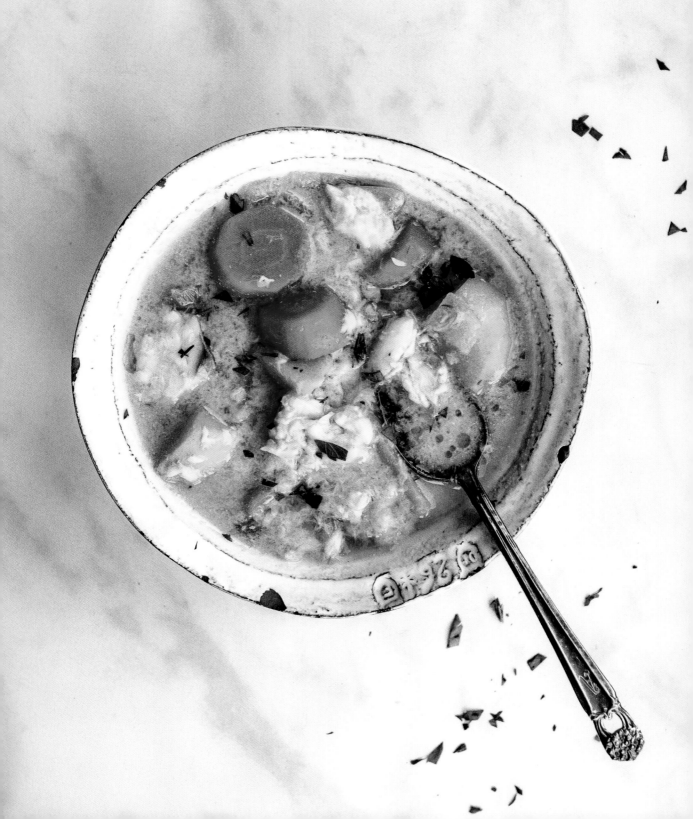

Lemony Greek Fisherman's Soup (*Psarosoupa*)

This light, fresh lemony soup has a homemade fish broth that is rich in marine collagen. It's hearty and reminiscent of a chowder because of the delicious *avgolemono*, or egg-lemon sauce. Adding egg yolks provides rich choline and other fabulous nutrients.

PREP TIME 10 minutes
COOK TIME 55 minutes
TOTAL TIME 1 hour and 5 minutes
YIELD 6 servings

SOUP

2 pounds (907 g) whole white fish with the head (red snapper or sea bass recommended), scaled and cleaned

8 cups (1.9 L) filtered water

1 teaspoon sea salt, divided

2 bay leaves

6–8 black peppercorns (omit for AIP)

¼ cup (59 ml) extra-virgin olive oil

1 small yellow onion, chopped

2 celery stalks, chopped

2 carrots, chopped

3 rutabagas, peeled and diced

½ teaspoon sea salt

¼ teaspoon black pepper (omit for AIP)

2 tablespoons (8 g) chopped parsley

EGG-LEMON SAUCE
(see note for AIP*)

2 egg yolks, room temperature

Juice of 1 lemon

½ tablespoon (5 g) arrowroot

To make the soup: Cut the fish in half widthwise (head on one piece, tail on the other). Place the water, fish, ½ teaspoon salt, bay leaves, and peppercorns in a large stockpot. Bring to a boil over medium-high heat, then reduce to a simmer. Cook, loosely covered, for 25 to 30 minutes. Skim off any scum that rises to the top with a slotted spoon.

Carefully transfer the fish to a platter. Strain the broth into a large pot. Discard the bay leaves. Rinse the pot and add the oil, onion, celery, and carrots. Cook over medium heat for 5 to 6 minutes, until the onions are soft. Add the broth, rutabagas, and salt. Simmer over medium heat for 15 to 20 minutes, until the rutabagas are fork-tender.

Separate the fish meat from the skin and bones, using your fingers to feel for small bones. Discard the skin, bones, and fish head, and cut the meat into bite-size pieces. Set aside.

To make the egg-lemon sauce: Whisk all the ingredients in a medium bowl until combined. Set aside.

Reduce the heat on the soup to medium-low. Whisk 1 to 2 cups (235 to 475 ml) of soup slowly into the bowl of egg-lemon sauce. This raises the temperature slowly and prevents it from turning into scrambled eggs! Pour the egg-lemon sauce into the soup. Stir well, letting it thicken the soup for 3 to 4 minutes over medium-low heat. Turn off the heat to let it continue thickening for 5 minutes, stirring occasionally.

Adjust the seasonings and lemon. Divide the fish among bowls and pour in the soup. Garnish with parsley. For leftovers, keep the fish separate from the soup and reheat with a little water or broth.

*For AIP, enjoy the Lemon Cream Sauce (page 112) in place of the Egg-Lemon Sauce.

Chicken Zoodle Soup

When I think of nourishing comfort food, I think of chicken zoodle soup. The homemade chicken stock has gut-soothing amino acids and is a staple in any "feel better" tool kit. Combined with tender veggies, oregano, and dill, it will warm your belly and soul.

PREP TIME 10 minutes

COOK TIME 1 hour and 15 minutes

TOTAL TIME 1 hour and 25 minutes

YIELD 4 to 6 servings

1 whole 3-pound (1.4-kg) chicken

½ teaspoon sea salt, plus more to taste

¼ teaspoon black pepper (omit for AIP)

2 medium yellow onions, peeled and cut into quarters

2 heads of garlic, cut in half widthwise to expose cloves

3–4 bay leaves

1–2 tablespoons (3–6 g) dried oregano, plus more to taste

3–4 tablespoons (12–16 g) chopped dill or 1 tablespoon (3 g) dried dill, plus more to taste

4 celery stalks, chopped, divided

4 carrots, chopped, divided

3½ quarts (3.3 L) filtered water

4 spiralized zucchinis or 4 servings of premade zoodles

Add the chicken, salt, pepper, onions, garlic, bay leaves, oregano, and dill to a large pot. Add half the celery and carrots. Pour water over everything; make sure it's enough to cover the chicken.

Bring to a low boil over medium-high heat and cook for about 30 minutes, until a thermometer inserted into the chicken reads 165°F (74°C). Gently remove the bird using 2 large spoons, being mindful of the water inside the cavity. Set the bird aside on a cutting board and let it rest for 3 to 5 minutes. Leave the water and veggies to continue cooking.

When cool enough to handle, peel the skin off the wings, breast, and drumsticks. Discard the skin.

Cut the breasts from the main carcass and leave them on your cutting board. Return the carcass, wings, and drumsticks to the water. Let simmer over medium-low heat for 40 minutes to create your stock.

Carefully remove the carcass and all chicken pieces. Place them onto your cutting board. Remove all the meat from the bones, shredding by hand or using 2 forks.

Turn the heat off. Carefully strain the chicken stock into another large pot using a fine-mesh strainer. Discard the veggies.

Return the chicken stock to your stovetop over low heat. Add the reserved carrots and celery and the meat on your cutting board to the freshly strained stock. Season to taste with salt, oregano, and/or dill. Add the zoodles and cook for 1 to 2 minutes.

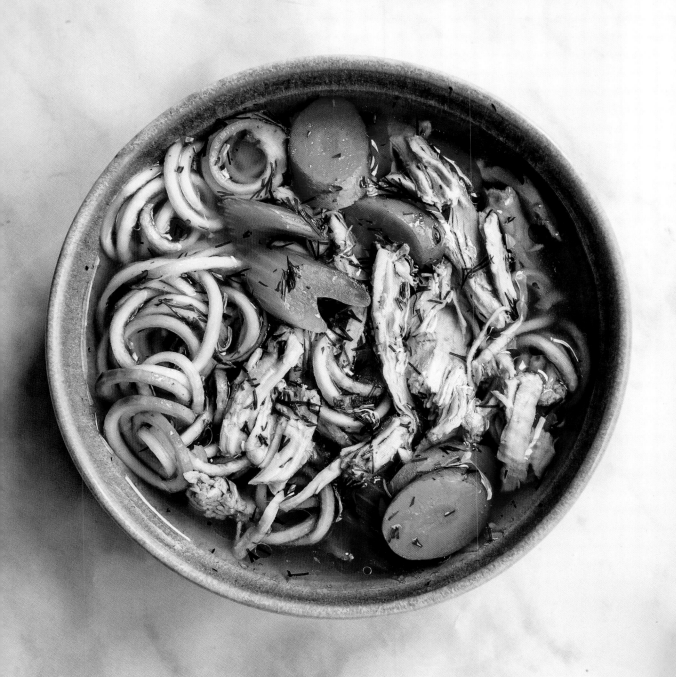

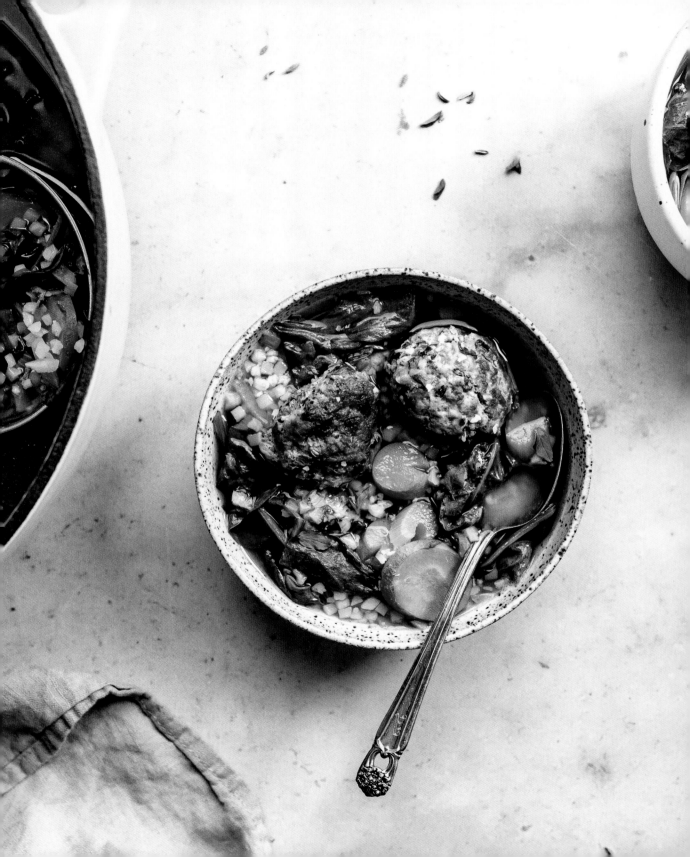

Italian Wedding Soup

This has always been one of my favorite soups! It's flavorful and the texture of it all is so comforting. You'll love this epic soup gone Paleo with cauliflower rice, homemade meatballs, and vegetables swimming around in bone broth.

PREP TIME 10 minutes
COOK TIME 45 minutes
TOTAL TIME 55 minutes
YIELD 4 servings

MEATBALLS

½ pound (225 g) ground pork

½ pound (225 g) grass-fed ground beef

½ tablespoon (2 g) chopped oregano or ½ teaspoon dried

¼ cup (15 g) chopped parsley or 3 teaspoons (4 g) dried

½ teaspoon fennel seeds or powder (omit for AIP)

2 teaspoons arrowroot or other Paleo-friendly flour

½ teaspoon sea salt

¼ teaspoon black pepper (omit for AIP)

1 tablespoon (15 ml) extra-virgin olive oil

SOUP

1 tablespoon (15 ml) of olive oil

2 carrots, chopped

1 small yellow onion, diced

3 celery stalks, chopped

4 cloves garlic, minced

6 cups (1.4 L) bone broth, store-bought or homemade (page 183)

¼ teaspoon sea salt

⅛ teaspoon black pepper (omit for AIP)

12 ounces (340 g) cauliflower rice

5 ounces (140 g) baby spinach

To make the meatballs: Combine beef and pork in a mixing bowl. Add the remaining ingredients except the oil, and mix by hand to combine well. Shape into small meatballs, about 1 inch (2.5 cm) each. Transfer them to a large plate, and set aside.

Heat the oil in a large Dutch oven over medium-high heat. Add the meatballs, turning occasionally on 2 or 3 sides, until cooked and browned. This should take 8 minutes; depending on the size of your pot, you may need to do this in batches.

Transfer meatballs to another plate while leaving the oil in your pot.

For the soup, add 1 tablespoon (15 ml) of oil to your pot over medium-high heat. Add the carrots, onion, and celery and sauté for 6 to 7 minutes, until softened. Add the garlic and sauté for 1 minute. Pour in the bone broth and season with salt and pepper.

Bring the soup to a boil, then add the cauliflower rice, meatballs, and baby spinach. Reduce the heat to medium-low, cover, and cook for 3 to 4 minutes, until the spinach is wilted and cauliflower rice is tender.

Creamy Ginger, Pear, and Butternut Squash Soup

Blending this soup makes it deliciously creamy, and the flavor is sweet, tangy, and savory. Enjoy it alone or add more protein, such as shredded chicken (page 74). Ginger is anti-inflammatory and has been shown to increase gut motility for smoother, more regular digestion. Combined with the fiber from the pears and rich bone broth, your gut will love this soothing soup.

PREP TIME 10 minutes
COOK TIME 45 minutes
TOTAL TIME 55 minutes
YIELD 4 servings

1 medium butternut squash, chopped into 1-inch (2.5-cm) cubes

1 large yellow onion, cut into 4 wedges

4 cloves garlic, whole and peeled

2 Bartlett or Bosch pears, cored and sliced into 4 wedges

3 tablespoons (45 ml) extra-virgin olive oil

¼ teaspoon sea salt, plus more to taste

⅛ teaspoon black pepper, plus more to taste (omit for AIP)

3½ cups (825 ml) bone broth, store-bought or homemade (page 183)

2 tablespoons plus ½ teaspoon (30 ml) ginger juice or 2 tablespoons (12 g) grated ginger

1 teaspoon ground turmeric

Fresh sprigs of thyme, sage, and toasted sesame seeds for garnish (optional; omit seeds for AIP)

Preheat the oven to 400°F (200°C, or gas mark 6). Line 2 baking sheets with parchment paper.

Toss the squash, onion, garlic, and pears with oil on the baking sheets. Sprinkle with salt and pepper. Roast in the oven for 30 to 35 minutes, until golden brown. Check midway and toss or rotate the pans to ensure everything is evenly cooked.

Add the bone broth to a large stockpot with the roasted vegetables. Bring to a boil, then reduce the heat to low and simmer for 15 minutes.

Turn off the heat. Add the ginger, turmeric, and more salt and pepper to taste and blend with an immersion blender. Alternatively, add everything to a blender. Blend until everything is well combined and the soup is smooth. Serve your soup in bowls with garnishes (if using).

Recipe Tip

Use frozen precut butternut squash to save time.

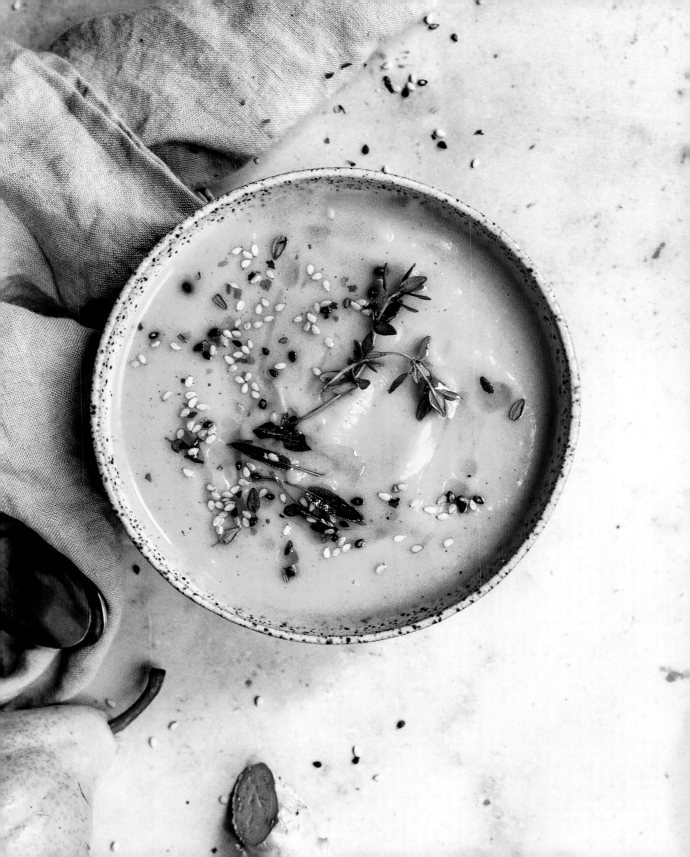

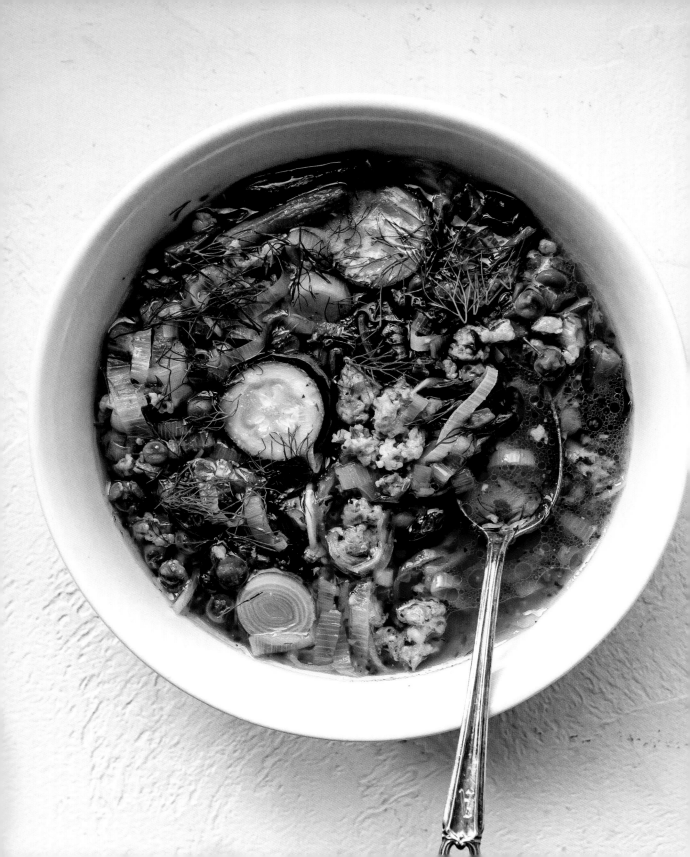

Green Minestrone Soup with Sausage

This spin on the traditional tomato-based minestrone uses all green vegetables and herbs. Adapt this herbaceous soup to any season. The variety of vegetables is great for your gut microbiome diversity, and it's benefiting your digestive health as you rotate in different foods to make variations.

PREP TIME 10 minutes
COOK TIME 20 minutes
TOTAL TIME 30 minutes
YIELD 4 to 6 servings

1 pound (454 g) ground pork or poultry

2 teaspoons ground fennel (omit for AIP)

1½ teaspoons dried oregano

1½ teaspoons dried parsley

1 teaspoon garlic powder

1 teaspoon onion powder

1 teaspoon dried basil

1¼ teaspoons sea salt, divided

1–2 tablespoons (15–30 ml) extra-virgin olive oil, divided (more oil if using ground poultry)

4 cloves garlic, sliced thinly

6 scallion stalks, chopped

Zest of 1 lemon

6 cups (1.4 L) chicken broth or chicken bone broth, store-bought or homemade (page 183)

2 leeks, chopped white and pale green parts, soaked in water

1 fennel, bulb and stalks, sliced thinly and fronds coarsely chopped

2 cups (248 g) green beans, trimmed and chopped (omit for AIP)

2 cups (240 g) chopped zucchini

2 cups (60 g) baby spinach or baby kale

1 cup (150 g) peas (omit for AIP)

1 tablespoon (15 ml) coconut aminos (optional)

4 lemon wedges (optional)

To a mixing bowl, add the meat, ground fennel, oregano, parsley, garlic powder, onion powder, basil, and 1 teaspoon of salt. Mix the seasonings well into the ground meat.

Heat a large stockpot over medium heat. Add 1 tablespoon (15 ml) of oil, and once shimmering, add the seasoned meat. Break up the meat as it cooks. Cook for 6 to 8 minutes, until starting to brown and the liquid released from the meat is absorbed. Remove the meat from the pot and set aside.

If using poultry, you may need to add 1 to 2 tablespoons (15 to 30 ml) of oil to the pot. Add the garlic, scallions, and zest. Stir for 5 to 7 minutes to meld with the fat, until the scallions soften

Add the broth. Raise the heat to medium-high, bringing to a simmer and stirring occasionally. Add the leeks, fennel bulb and stalks, green beans, and zucchini. Reduce the heat to medium. Season with ¼ teaspoon of salt. Cook for 5 to 7 minutes, stirring occasionally.

When the vegetables are fork-tender, add the ground meat, spinach, peas, and coconut aminos (if using), stirring for 20 seconds, until the spinach is wilted and peas are bright green.

Divide the soup into bowls, top with fennel fronds, and serve with lemon wedges (if using).

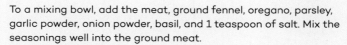

Make It AIP

Omit the fennel seeds (fresh fennel is okay), green beans, and peas. Add more zucchini and spinach, or add some carrots or other quick-cooking vegetables.

Bone Broth Ramen

This easy, throw-together meal is nourishing and tastes like it's been cooking all day long. With the right prep, you'll have it together in no time. For those healing their gut in conjunction with a thyroid condition, iodine from the nori (seaweed) is a very supportive nutrient.

PREP TIME 15 minutes
COOK TIME 10 minutes
TOTAL TIME 25 minutes
YIELD 4 servings

4 packages (4 ounces, or 115 g each) of shirataki or kelp noodles (sub veggie noodles for AIP)

1 tablespoon (15 ml) extra-virgin olive oil

2 cups (140 g) sliced mixed mushrooms

6 cups (1.4 L) bone broth, store-bought or homemade (page 183)

2 tablespoons (28 ml) coconut aminos

1 tablespoon (15 ml) ginger juice or 3 tablespoons (18 g) minced ginger

3 scallions, chopped

4 cups (120 g) baby spinach or baby kale

1 teaspoon toasted sesame oil (omit for AIP)

16 ounces (455 g) or 4 slices of prepared garlic pulled pork (pernil, page 77)

2 carrots, sliced thinly into matchsticks or 1 cup (110 g) shredded carrots

2 soft-boiled eggs (omit for AIP)

8 nori sheet slices (plain)

Microgreens and/or toasted sesame seeds (optional, omit seeds for AIP)

Rinse the shirataki noodles well in a fine-mesh strainer with water for 30 seconds. Let drain over a bowl

To a large stockpot, add the oil over medium-high heat. Once shimmering, add the mushrooms and sauté for 3 to 5 minutes, until soft. Remove the mushrooms from the pot and set aside.

To the pot, add bone broth, coconut aminos, ginger, scallions, and shirataki noodles (or veggie noodles that need to be cooked, such as sweet potato noodles). Bring it all to a simmer over medium heat. Add the spinach and stir in until wilted.

Turn the heat off and drizzle with toasted sesame oil. Mix in well and adjust to taste. Using tongs, add the noodles and wilted greens to large serving bowls. Pour the remaining heated broth over the top of each bowl. Layer in the mushrooms, pork, carrots, and half a boiled egg to each bowl, and tuck the nori sheets in the side of the bowl. Garnish as desired with microgreens or sesame seeds.

Recipe Tip

Substitute shredded chicken if you'd like. Pork is more traditional, but I'll throw anything I have in here. Make use of what you have in the fridge.

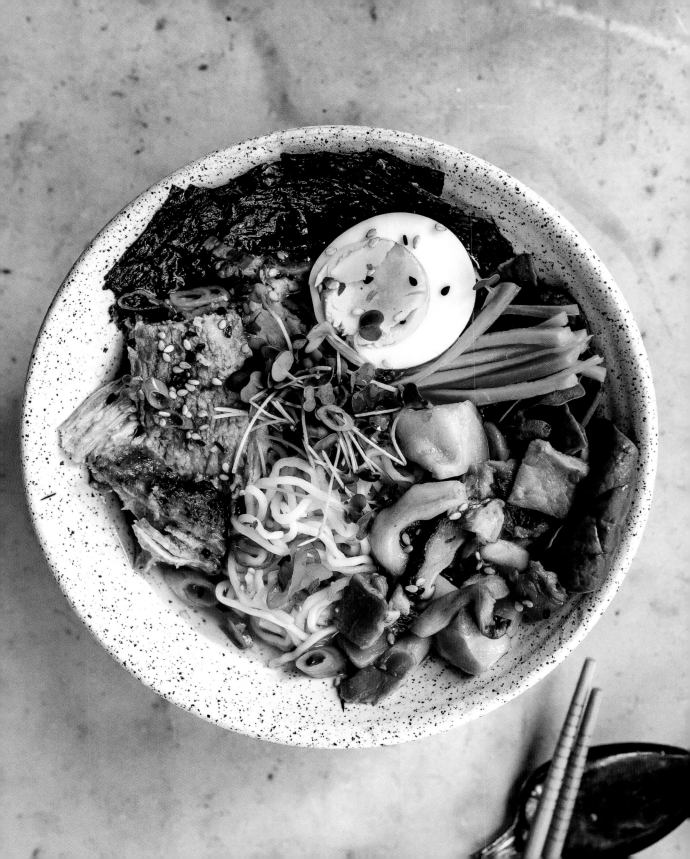

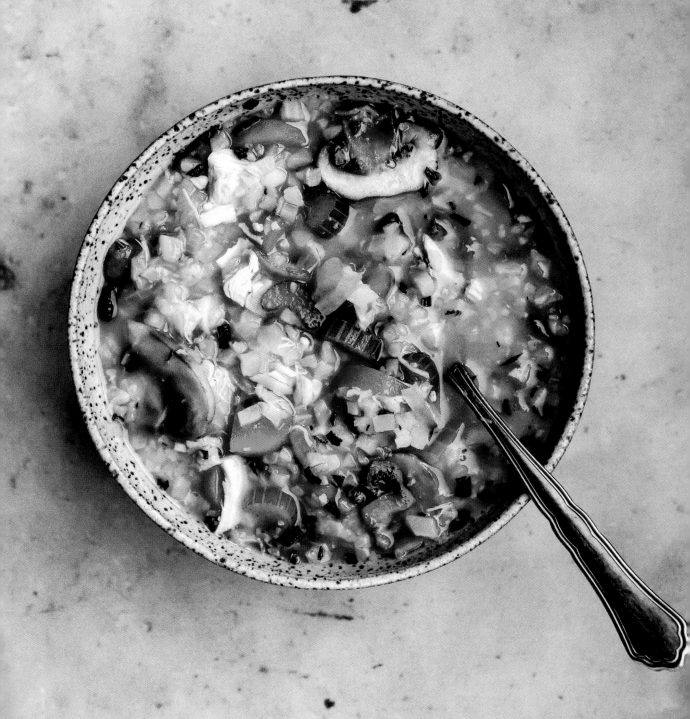

Mushroom and Cauliflower Rice Soup with Chicken

If you're a mushroom-and-rice soup lover, this soup is so satisfying. Cauliflower rice gives you a similar mouthfeel, and the sweet potato cream sauce adds richness. It comes together in a flash because we're using prepared chicken and broth. Leftovers from the Spatchcock Chicken and Artichokes (page 91) would be great, or use a store-bought rotisserie chicken or the Instant Pot Shredded Chicken (page 74).

PREP TIME 10 minutes
COOK TIME 25 minutes
TOTAL TIME 35 minutes
YIELD 4 to 6 servings

1 white sweet potato, peeled and diced

4–5 cups (940 ml to 1.2 L) filtered water, divided

1 tablespoon (15 ml) extra-virgin olive oil

3 medium carrots, chopped

3 celery stalks, chopped

8 ounces (225 g) cremini mushrooms, sliced

½ yellow onion, chopped

3 cloves garlic, minced

4 cups (940 ml) basic broth or bone broth, store-bought or homemade (page 183)

1 teaspoon sea salt

½ tablespoon (1 g) chopped rosemary or ¼ teaspoon dried rosemary, crushed

½ tablespoon (1¼ g) chopped sage or ¼ teaspoon dried sage

½ tablespoon (2 g) chopped thyme or ¼ teaspoon dried thyme

¼ teaspoon black pepper (omit for AIP)

2 chicken breasts, cooked and shredded

16 ounces (455 g) fresh or frozen cauliflower rice

Add the sweet potato to a pot with 2 cups (475 ml) of water or more to cover. Boil for 10 to 12 minutes, until fork-tender. Drain and add it to a blender with 1 to 2 cups (235 to 475 ml) of water to form a cream sauce. You want a loose puree, similar to the consistency of soup. It should yield 2 cups (475 ml); adjust the water as needed. Set aside.

To a large stockpot, add the oil over medium heat. Once shimmering, add carrots, celery, mushrooms, and onion. Stir for 5 to 6 minutes, until the onion and mushrooms are softened. Stir in the garlic for 30 seconds.

Pour the broth on top of vegetables and add all the seasonings. Simmer for 10 to 12 minutes, until the veggies are tender.

Add the shredded chicken and cauliflower rice. Stir to combine. Add the 2 cups (475 ml) of potato puree and stir in well to create a creamy soup. Remove from the heat and serve!

Recipe Tip

The white sweet potato puree or "cream sauce" can be made in advance.

Instant Pot Beef Stew

I make this beef stew recipe almost weekly in the cold months . . . and sometimes in the warm months, too. We're that obsessed with it! It's always comforting, nourishing, and easy to throw together. Using bone broth or basic broth here is a great way to get a little dose of broth. Go on and double the batch for leftovers!

PREP TIME 10 minutes
COOK TIME 1 hour
TOTAL TIME 1 hour and 10 minutes
YIELD 4 servings

2 tablespoons (30 ml) extra-virgin olive oil

1–1½ pounds (455–680 g) beef chuck/stew meat, cut in 2-inch (5-cm) chunks

¼ teaspoon sea salt, plus more to taste

¼ teaspoon black pepper (omit for AIP)

3 medium carrots, cut into 3-inch (7.5-cm) slices

1 large yellow onion, cut in wedges

3 cloves garlic, minced

3 large sprigs of thyme, divided

1 tablespoon (9 g) arrowroot

1 tablespoon (15 ml) balsamic vinegar

1½–2 cups (355–475 ml) bone broth, store-bought or homemade (page 183)

2 rutabagas or turnips, cut into quarters

2 bay leaves or 2 teaspoons crushed bay leaves

Add the oil to your Instant Pot on the Sauté mode. Once sizzling, add the meat and brown for 5 to 8 minutes, seasoning with salt and pepper. This is your chance to get it brown on all sides. Flip as needed with a wooden spoon, but not too often, so it can get a nice color and crust on the exterior. When the meat is finished and all liquid is absorbed, place it in a bowl and set aside.

Add the carrots, onion, garlic, and 2 sprigs of thyme to the pot. Sauté for 2 to 3 minutes, scraping the brown bits from the meat with a wooden spoon. Add the arrowroot and stir well. Add the vinegar, broth, meat, rutabagas, remaining thyme, and bay leaves with a pinch of salt on top. Press everything down with a wooden spoon; it's okay if not everything is submerged.

Close the lid on the Instant Pot and close the steam valve. Press the meat/stew button, or set the cooker to 35 minutes of high pressure. After 35 minutes of high pressure, allow the cooker to naturally cool and release pressure for 15 to 20 minutes. If you're in a rush, carefully do a quick release after 5 to 10 minutes.

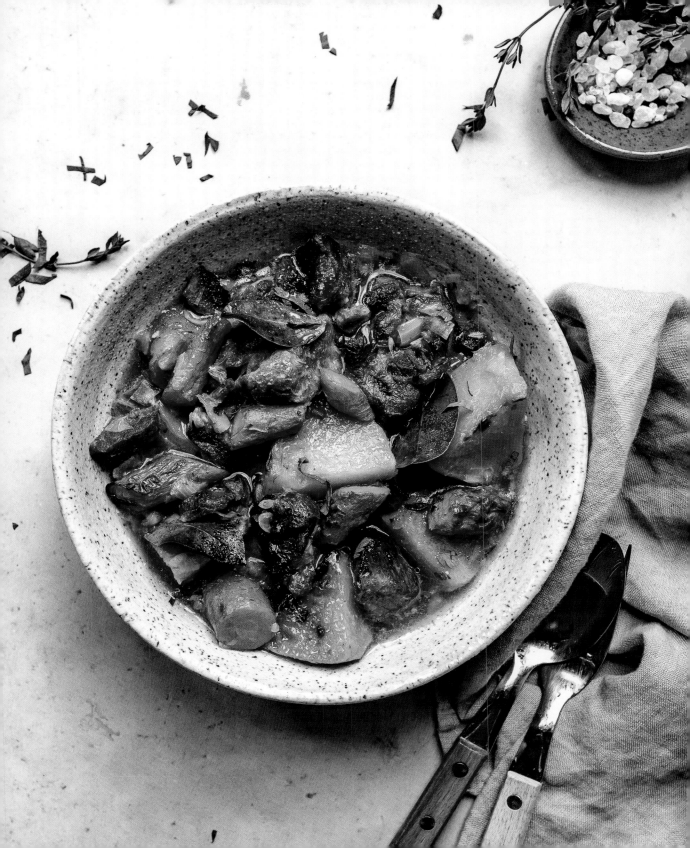

Instant Pot Shredded Chicken

Having ready-to-go shredded chicken in your fridge during the week is a major lifesaver. You'll find so many ways to use it cold or hot and just in life! Try it in the Massaged Kale Caesar (page 140). Flavor it with your favorite dried herbs. I keep it simple here so it can be used in any recipe.

PREP TIME 5 minutes
COOK TIME 20 minutes
TOTAL TIME 25 minutes
YIELD 4 to 8 servings

4 large chicken breasts, skinless and boneless (2½ to 3 pounds, or 1.1 to 1.3 kg (boneless optional)

½ cup (120 ml) bone broth (page 183), broth, or filtered water

1 teaspoon sea salt

Add the chicken breasts, broth, and salt to the Instant Pot. Try to keep the chicken in a single layer, or close to it, for even cooking. Place the lid on and turn the valve to "sealing." Pressure cook on high for 10 minutes, followed by a 5- to 10-minute natural release. Carefully turn valve to "venting" and remove the lid with an oven mitt.

Remove the chicken breasts using tongs and place them in a large mixing bowl. Using 2 forks, shred the chicken breast. You can season the chicken more here or even add a favorite sauce

To store, add your shredded chicken to an airtight container and pour over at least half of the liquid so it will stay moist. This can stay stored in the refrigerator for up to 5 days or frozen for 1 month.

Instant Pot Lamb Shanks

Lamb shanks are a notoriously tough cut. You have to braise them for a long time to get them tender and falling off the bone. Thanks to electric pressure cookers, we can cut that time significantly! Serve these with a mashed cauliflower to drench in sauce.

PREP TIME 10 minutes

COOK TIME 1 hour and 40 minutes

TOTAL TIME 1 hour and 50 minutes

YIELD 4 servings

2–3 lamb shanks

½ teaspoon sea salt

¼ teaspoon black pepper (omit for AIP)

1½ tablespoons (23 ml) extra-virgin olive oil, divided

1 yellow onion, diced

2 large carrots, sliced ½ inch (1 cm) thick

3 tablespoons (27 g) arrowroot

1½ cups (355 ml) bone broth, store-bought or homemade (page 183)

3 tablespoons (45 ml) balsamic vinegar

1 tablespoon (15 ml) coconut aminos

7 ounces (196 g) tomato puree (sub sweet potato puree for AIP)

1 tablespoon (16 g) tomato paste (omit for AIP)

3 cloves garlic, minced

½ tablespoon (1 g) chopped rosemary

2 tablespoons (8 g) chopped parsley, divided

2 bay leaves

Mashed cauliflower (page 125) or veggie confetti rice (page 133)

Set the Instant Pot to sauté. While it heats up, wash and pat dry lamb shanks with a paper towel, and trim any excess fat. Season the lamb shanks with salt and pepper on all sides.

When the pot is hot, add ½ tablespoon (8 g) of oil. Sear 2 shanks in the hot oil, until browned on all sides. Repeat with any remaining shanks and an additional ½ tablespoon (8 g) of oil. Set the browned shanks aside on a plate.

Add the remaining oil to the pot and sauté the onion and carrots for 3 to 4 minutes, until the onion softens. Stir in the arrowroot. Add the broth, vinegar, coconut aminos, tomato puree, tomato paste, garlic, rosemary, 1 tablespoon (4 g) parsley, and bay leaves. Stir well, scraping up any bits from the bottom.

Add the lamb shanks back to the pot, nestling them with the vegetables in the liquid. Cover and lock the lid into place. Set to manual or meat/stew mode. Choose high pressure for 75 minutes of cook time.

After cooking, carefully turn the valve to release the steam with an oven mitt or allow it to release slowly for 10 minutes.

Remove the lamb shanks from the pot and plate them. Set the Instant Pot to sear or sauté. Stir well and allow the sauce to thicken uncovered for 5 minutes.

Pour the finished sauce over your lamb shanks. Garnish with remaining parsley, and serve with mashed cauliflower or veggie rice.

Recipe Tip

Got leftover sauce? I love using it for pulled chicken or meatballs!

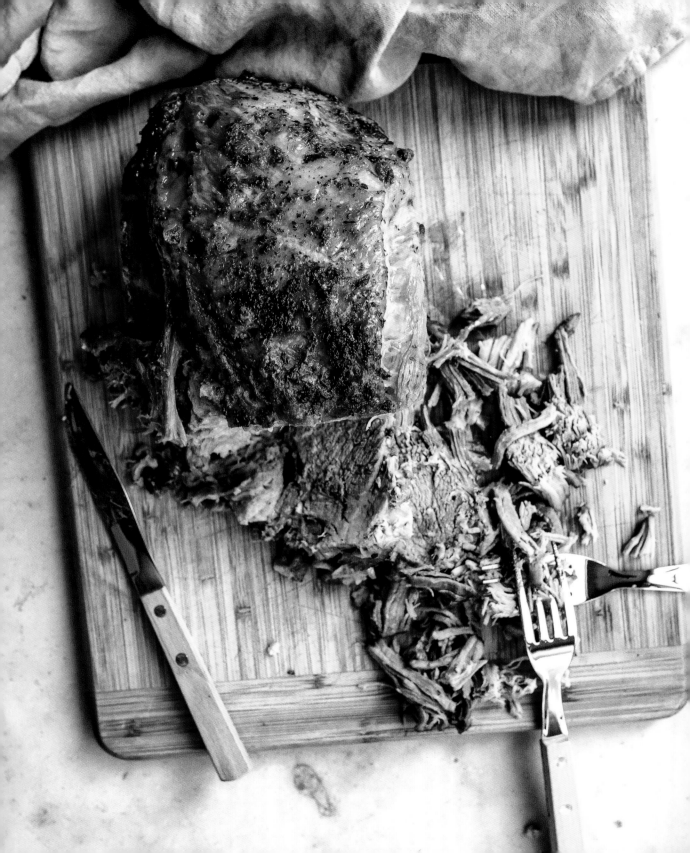

Instant Pot Pernil *(Garlic Pulled Pork)*

Every Christmas Eve, my grandparents would make *pernil*, a traditional Puerto Rican garlic pork dish. I have happy memories of my grandfather marinating a pork butt for twenty-four hours, then cooking it all day long while we gathered presents under the tree. This dish and my grandmother's coquito (coconut eggnog)—nothing beats it! But why wait for garlic pork goodness? I love using my Instant Pot to make this flavorful dish all year round and serving it with cauliflower rice and tostones (page 118).

PREP TIME 1 to 24 hours
COOK TIME 1 hour and 40 minutes
TOTAL TIME 3+ hours
YIELD 4 servings

7–8 cloves garlic, minced

½ tablespoon (9 g) sea salt

1½ teaspoons black pepper (omit for AIP)

½ tablespoon (2 g) dried oregano

¼ cup (59 ml) extra-virgin olive oil

1 pork butt (shoulder), 3–4 lb., or 1.4–1.8 kg

4 bay leaves

¼ cup (60 ml) bone broth (store-bought or homemade, page 183) or water

In a bowl, mix the garlic, salt, pepper, oregano, and oil to form a paste.

Remove any "silver skin" or any skin from the pork butt, but leave the layer of fat on. Add the pork to another large bowl. Poke the roast all over with a small paring knife to make several slits.

Rub the garlic paste all over the pork and into the crevices and slits so it's well coated. Cover the bowl with aluminum foil and let marinate in the refrigerator for at least 1 hour and up to 24 hours.

Place the pork butt in your Instant Pot (on the rack if you have it). Add the bay leaves and pour bone broth in the bottom. Set your Instant Pot to the meat/stew option for 70 minutes and let it naturally release for 15 minutes.

Line a baking sheet with parchment paper. Turn your oven broiler on and arrange a rack low in the oven to fit the pork butt in. Turn the Instant Pot valve carefully using an oven mitt. Open the lid and using tongs or large spoons add the pork butt to the baking sheet. Discard the bay leaves and reserve the broth/juices in a small bowl.

Broil the pork for 5 to 10 minutes to get crispy. The fat layer should be golden brown and bubbling along with the meat when done. Watch it closely so it doesn't burn and remove when desired. The internal temperature should be at least 145°F (63°C) when checked with a meat thermometer.

Remove from the oven and let rest for 10 minutes to keep the meat moist. Cut or shred the meat and pour the juices over top. Save leftovers in an airtight container for up to 5 days.

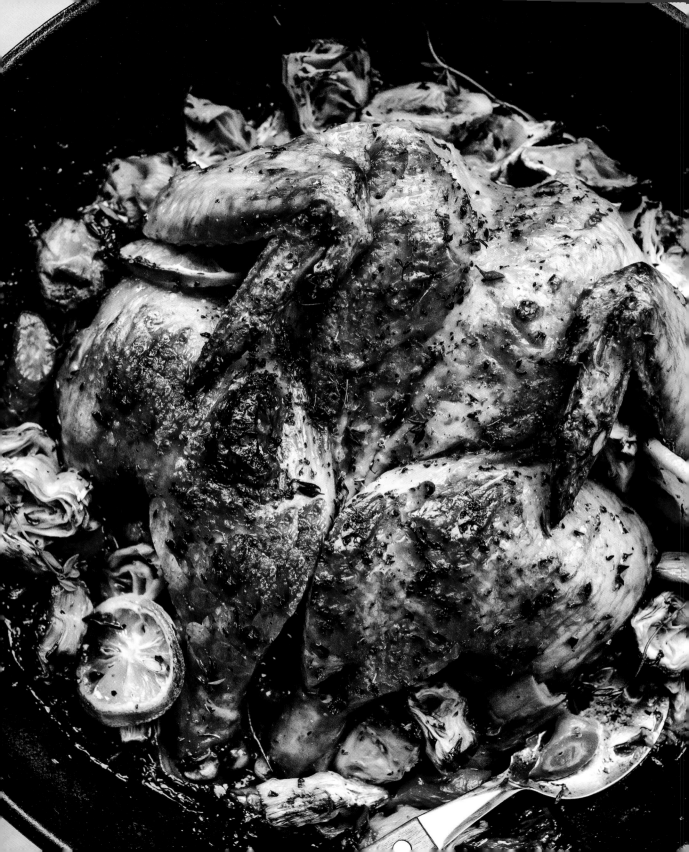

4

ENTRÉES

Eating Paleo or AIP never stops me (and my eclectic palate) from enjoying something I love. Inspired by my culture and my husband's, our favorite restaurant dishes, and our travels, I re-create dishes we enjoy—with plenty of vitamin J. (Joy, obviously.) Invite your family and friends because even the picky eaters will love these main dishes.

Picadillo with Plantain Rice 80

Chicken Marbella 83

Chicken, Bacon, Brussels Sprouts, and Squash Skillet 84

Green Goddess Skillet 87

Creamy Chicken and Mushroom Risotto 88

Lemon Spatchcock Chicken and Artichokes 91

Crispy Golden Salmon 92

Meat Hash with Kale and Cabbage 94

Herb-Stuffed Frittata 95

Rib Eye Steak with Chimichurri 97

"Cheesesteak" Stuffed Sweet Potatoes 98

Crispy Roasted Chicken Thighs with Salsa Verde 100

Sweet-and-Sour Meatballs with Roasted Cauliflower 101

Teriyaki Salmon and Bok Choy 102

Shrimp and Broccoli 103

Mango Chicken Jibaritos (*Plantain Sandwiches*) 105

Pastelón (*Puerto Rican Casserole*) 106

Spaghetti Squash Pastitsio (*Greek Baked Ziti*) 108

Moussaka (*Greek Eggplant Casserole*) 109

Creamy Chicken and Broccoli Bake 111

Greek Stuffed Cabbage Rolls in Lemony Sauce 112

Pesto Primavera Veggie Noodles with Shrimp 115

Picadillo with Plantain Rice

This Puerto Rican hash is filled with delicious spices, sweet raisins, and salty and briny olives. I grew up eating it over white rice with *platanos*, or plantains—either sweet *maduros* or salty *tostones* (page 118). Here I decided to be cheeky and have it over plantain rice instead! Use green plantains. If you use a ripe yellow plantain or leave the seeds in, the plantains won't rice well and will stick together.

PREP TIME 10 minutes
COOK TIME 45 minutes
TOTAL TIME 55 minutes
YIELD 4 servings

PLANTAIN RICE
2 medium green (unripe) plantains

1 tablespoon (14 g) coconut oil

2 tablespoons (28 ml) basic broth or bone broth (store-bought or homemade, page 182 or 183) or water

¼ teaspoon sea salt

PICADILLO
1 medium yellow onion, finely chopped

2 tablespoons (30 ml) extra-virgin olive oil

2 cloves garlic, minced

1 pound (454 g) ground meat (beef or bison recommended)

¼ teaspoon sea salt

¼ teaspoon black pepper (optional; omit for AIP)

2 teaspoons dried oregano

1 teaspoon ground cumin (sub with cinnamon for AIP)

3–4 tablespoons (3–4 g) chopped cilantro, plus more for garnish

2–3 tablespoons (32–48 g) tomato paste (optional; omit or sub for AIP)

¼ cup (60 ml) bone broth, store-bought or homemade (page 183)

⅓ cup (33 g) chopped green pitted olives

¼ cup (35 g) raisins

To make the plantain rice: Cut the ends off the plantains, then cut them in half widthwise and lengthwise. Peel the skin off. With a spoon, scoop out and discard the soft center with the seeds. Slice the plantains into matchsticks and add them to a food processor. Pulse lightly, until rice forms.

In a nonstick skillet with a lid, heat the coconut oil over medium-high heat. Add your rice and stir it. Let it get golden brown for 4 to 5 minutes. Add the broth and salt, reduce the heat to low, and cover. Let it steam/simmer for 10 minutes. Fluff with a fork and set aside.

To make the picadillo: Over medium heat, sauté the onion in the oil for 8 to 10 minutes, until soft and translucent. Add the garlic and stir with a wooden spoon for 30 seconds. Add the ground meat, breaking it up with the wooden spoon. Season with salt and pepper (if using). Add the oregano, cumin, and cilantro. Keep breaking up the meat with your wooden spoon as the meat cooks, until most of the pink is gone. Stir in the tomato paste (if using) and your broth. Mix very well so the paste doesn't get clumpy.

Let simmer for 10 minutes, stirring occasionally. Add the olives and raisins, and let simmer for 10 minutes. Taste to adjust any seasonings as you'd like! Turn off the heat, sprinkle with some cilantro, and serve over plantain rice.

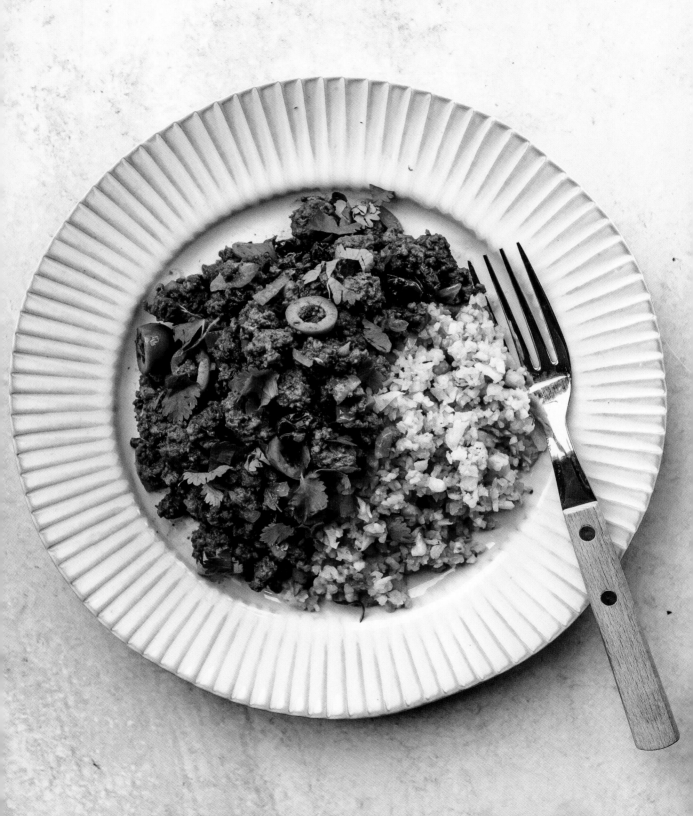

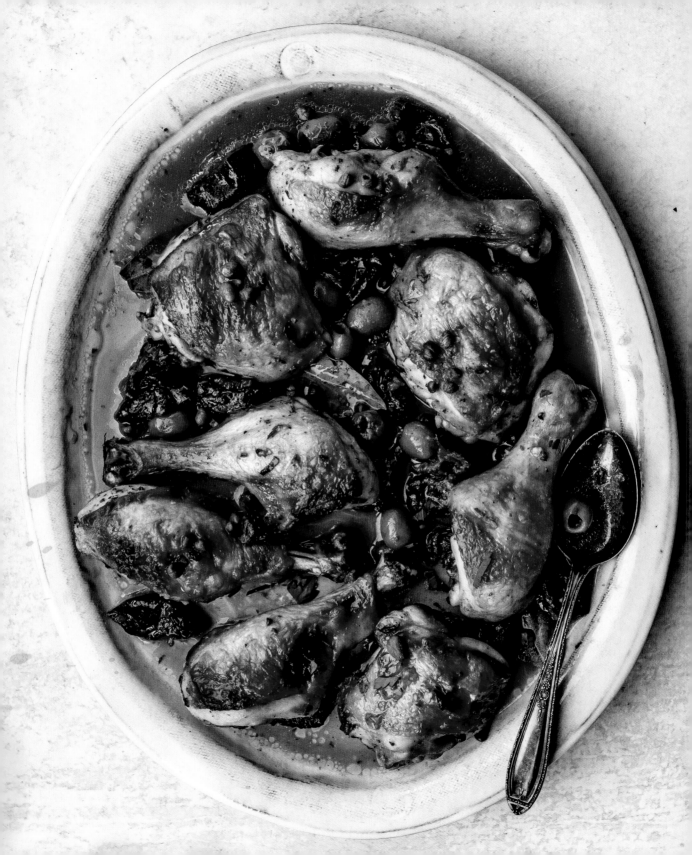

Chicken Marbella

This nostalgic dish has been Paleo-fied from *The Silver Palate Cookbook*. It originally called for white wine and brown sugar. Use vinegar, a little lemon juice, and raw honey with broth to make the epic marinade sauce that's sweet and briny from the prunes, olives, and capers. This is delicious served over sautéed spinach or a nice green salad with a forkful of Fermented Coleslaw (page 184).

PREP TIME 2 to 24 hours
COOK TIME 45 minutes
TOTAL TIME 2+ hours
YIELD 4 servings

¼ cup (59 ml) extra-virgin olive oil

¼ cup (60 ml) red wine vinegar

⅓ cup (58 g) pitted prunes

½ cup (50 g) green pitted olives

2 tablespoons (18 g) capers with brine (for AIP, use AIP-compliant capers without citric acid or distilled vinegar)

4 bay leaves

4 cloves garlic, minced

1 tablespoon (3 g) dried oregano

½ teaspoon ground cinnamon

1½ teaspoons sea salt, divided

¼ teaspoon black pepper (omit for AIP)

4 pounds (1.8 kg) bone-in chicken drumsticks and thighs with skin

2 tablespoons (40 g) raw honey

Juice of 1 lemon

1 cup (235 ml) chicken broth or chicken bone broth, store-bought or homemade (page 183)

Combine the oil, vinegar, prunes, olives, capers, bay leaves, garlic, oregano, cinnamon, ½ teaspoon salt, and pepper in a bowl. Add cleaned chicken pieces to it. Toss the chicken to coat in the marinade. Cover tightly and marinate in the refrigerator for at least 2 hours and up to overnight.

Preheat the oven to 375°F (190°C, or gas mark 5). To a roasting pan, add the chicken (skin-side up) and marinade in one layer. Season with 1 teaspoon of salt.

Whisk the honey, lemon juice, and broth in a mixing bowl. Pour it around the chicken. Roast chicken for 45 minutes, until the internal temperature is 165°F (74°C).

Optionally broil the chicken for 3 to 5 minutes, if you'd like more crisp skin! Serve the chicken, prunes, and olives with your pan sauce.

Chicken, Bacon, Brussels Sprouts, and Squash Skillet

Who can turn down a sweet and savory veggie-packed chicken dish? And a one-pan wonder, no less? Make a double batch for ample leftovers, because this one will be devoured fast . . . trust me.

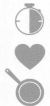

PREP TIME 10 minutes
COOK TIME 30 minutes
TOTAL TIME 40 minutes
YIELD 4 servings

2 large skinless chicken breasts or 4 skinless chicken cutlets, cleaned and cut into small ½-inch (1-cm) pieces (about 1½ cups, or 210 g)

¼ teaspoon sea salt

¼ teaspoon black pepper (omit for AIP)

6 slices of nitrite-free bacon, chopped

1 small-medium butternut squash, peeled and cubed into small pieces as shown (or 1½ cups, or 210 g, precubed)

12 ounces (340 g) Brussels sprouts, chopped into thirds

¼ cup bone broth, store-bought or homemade (page 183) or water

Season the chicken with salt and pepper. Set aside.

Add the bacon to a large cast-iron skillet over medium heat. Toss with a wooden spoon for 5 to 7 minutes, until the fat renders and bacon is cooked. Remove the bacon from the pan and set aside.

Add the chicken to the bacon fat in the pan. Cook for 6 minutes, stirring, until golden. Add it to the same plate as your bacon bits. Using the same pan, add your vegetables, and stir well to coat. Cook on the stove top for 5 minutes, then add your cooking liquid. Stir and reduce the heat to medium-low. Cover the pan with a lid and let cook for 10 to 12 minutes, until the vegetables are fork-tender.

Most or all liquid should be absorbed into the veggies. Add chicken and bacon back to the pan and stir to heat through.

Recipe Tip

Substitute sweet potato for the butternut squash, if needed.

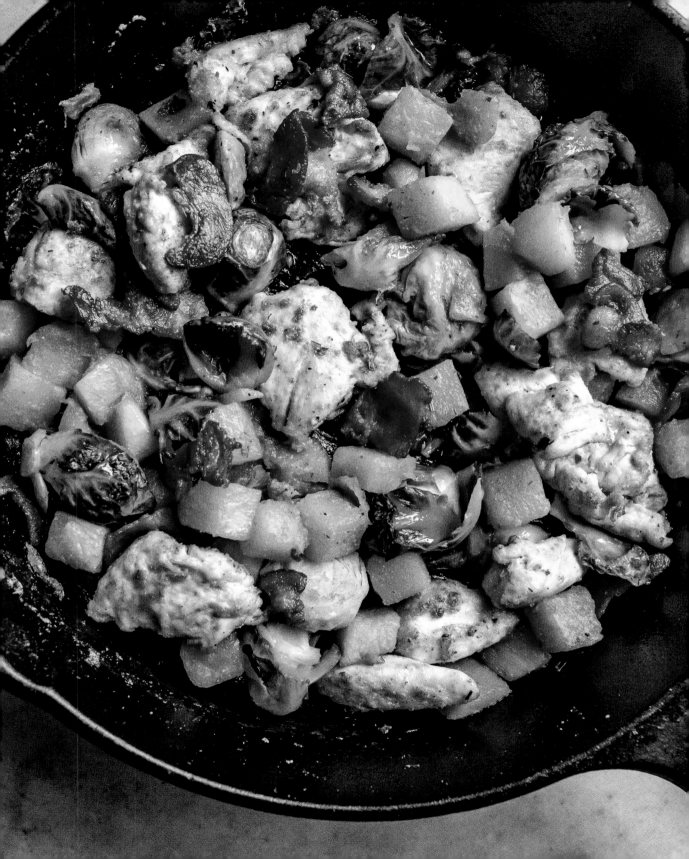

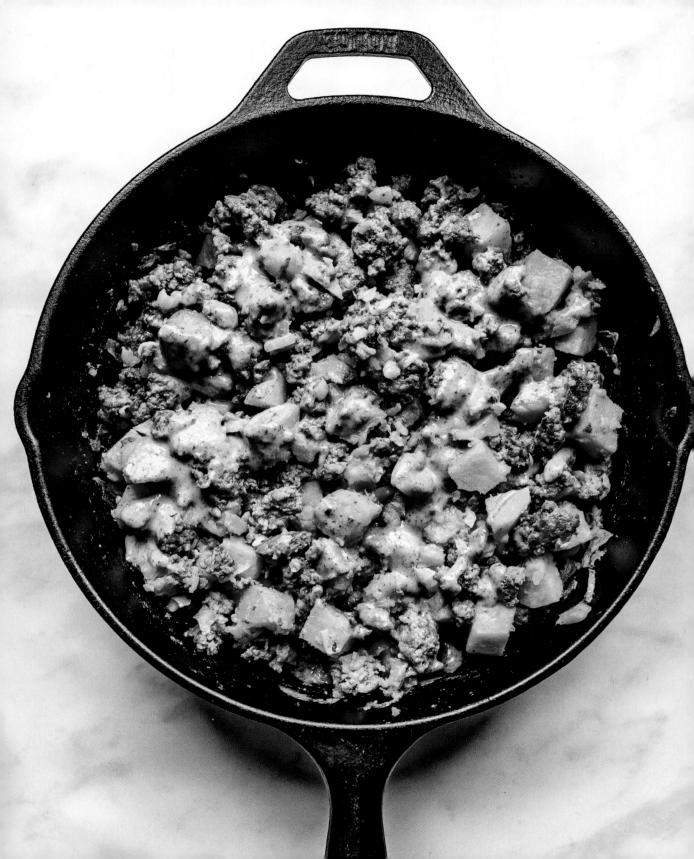

Green Goddess Skillet

This colorful skillet is another ground meat wonder that is bursting with flavor, veggies, and herbs. It is easy enough to throw together in one pan on a weeknight. It also makes a great batch meal; just hold the dressing and serve it on the side.

PREP TIME 10 minutes
COOK TIME 25 minutes
TOTAL TIME 35 minutes
YIELD 4 servings

GREEN GODDESS DRESSING
¼ cup (60 g) unsweetened coconut yogurt (homemade, page 187, or additive-free if store-bought) or avocado

¼ cup (12 g) basil leaves

¼ cup (12 g) chopped chives

Juice of ½ lemon

½ teaspoon apple cider vinegar

⅓ cup (80 ml) coconut milk (additive-free, water and coconut only)

SKILLET
2 tablespoons (30 ml) extra-virgin olive oil

1 pound (454 g) grass-fed ground beef, bison, or free-range ground poultry

½ small yellow onion, diced

1 small clove garlic, minced

1½ cups (165 g) diced sweet potato

¼ teaspoon sea salt

⅛ teaspoon black pepper (omit for AIP)

¼ cup (60 ml) water or bone broth, store-bought or homemade (page 183)

To make the dressing: Add all the ingredients to a food processor. Pulse until smooth. Set aside in an airtight container. This will store well in the fridge for 7 to 8 days.

To make the skillet: Heat the oil in a large cast-iron skillet over medium-high heat. Add the meat and cook for 5 minutes, using a wooden spoon to break it up and mix. Add the onion and garlic, stirring as the meat browns. Cook for 4 to 5 minutes, until the onion is soft. Add the sweet potato, and season with salt and pepper.

Reduce the heat to medium-low, and add the water. Cover the skillet with a lid and let cook for 15 to 20 minutes, until potatoes are fork-tender. Remove the skillet from heat and drizzle with the dressing.

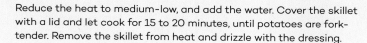

Creamy Chicken and Mushroom Risotto

Making traditional risotto can be intimidating, but when you're just using cauliflower rice, veggies, and ground meat . . . it's a breeze and still made with lots of love. Try mixing in a dollop of Instant Pot Coconut Yogurt (page 187) for creaminess and probiotics.

PREP TIME 5 minutes
COOK TIME 35 minutes
TOTAL TIME 40 minutes
YIELD 4 servings

SWEET POTATO PUREE
(yields about 3½ cups, or 788 g)

1½–2 cups (165–220 g) peeled and diced white sweet potato

3–4 cups (708–940 ml) filtered water, divided

TOPPING "PEPITASAN"
(yields about ½ cup, or 50g)

⅓ cup (47 g) pepitas (preferably sprouted; omit for AIP)

½ teaspoon sea salt

¼ teaspoon garlic powder

1 tablespoon (5 g) nutritional yeast

RISOTTO
4 tablespoons (52 g) ghee (sub olive oil for AIP replacement), divided

1 pound (454 g) ground chicken

2 teaspoons sea salt, divided

½ teaspoon black pepper, divided (omit for AIP)

½ teaspoon garlic powder, divided

2 shallots or 1 small yellow onion, chopped

8 ounces (225 g) cremini mushrooms, sliced

5 ounces (140 g) mixed mushrooms, sliced

5 ounces (140 g) baby spinach

16 ounces (455 g) cauliflower rice

½ cup (120 ml) basic or bone broth (pages 182 or 183)

To make the puree: Boil the sweet potato in a pot with enough water to cover, until fork-tender. Drain and add the potatoes to a blender with 1 cup (235 ml) of water. Blend to form a cream sauce similar to a pumpkin puree. Add more water, if needed. Set aside.

To make the topping: Add all of the ingredients to a food processor or grinder. Pulse until well combined. Taste and adjust seasonings. Set aside.

To make the risotto: Heat 1 tablespoon (13 g) of ghee in a deep skillet over medium heat. Add the chicken, ½ teaspoon salt, ¼ teaspoon pepper, and ¼ teaspoon garlic powder. Break up the meat with a wooden spoon. Cook for 6 to 7 minutes, until cooked through. Transfer to a plate and set aside.

Add 1 tablespoon of ghee and the shallots to the skillet and cook for 3 minutes. Add 1 tablespoon of ghee and the mushrooms and cook for 3 to 4 minutes. Stir in the baby spinach, salt, pepper, and remaining garlic powder. Cook for 2 minutes, until the greens are wilted. The mushroom liquid should be reabsorbed before moving on. Transfer half the vegetables to a plate and set aside.

Add 1 tablespoon of ghee, the cauliflower rice, and chicken to the skillet. Mix well and cook for 3 minutes. Add ½ cup (113 g) of puree and stir until combined. Slowly pour in ¼ cup (60 ml) of broth.

Bring to a low simmer and cook, until you have a creamy risotto-like consistency. Lower the heat and add more puree to thicken or broth to loosen. Cook for 3 to 4 minutes, until the liquid absorbs into the cauliflower and meat.

Top the risotto with the vegetables and a few tablespoons of pepitasan. Store the pepitasan in an airtight container in the refrigerator for up to 1 month.

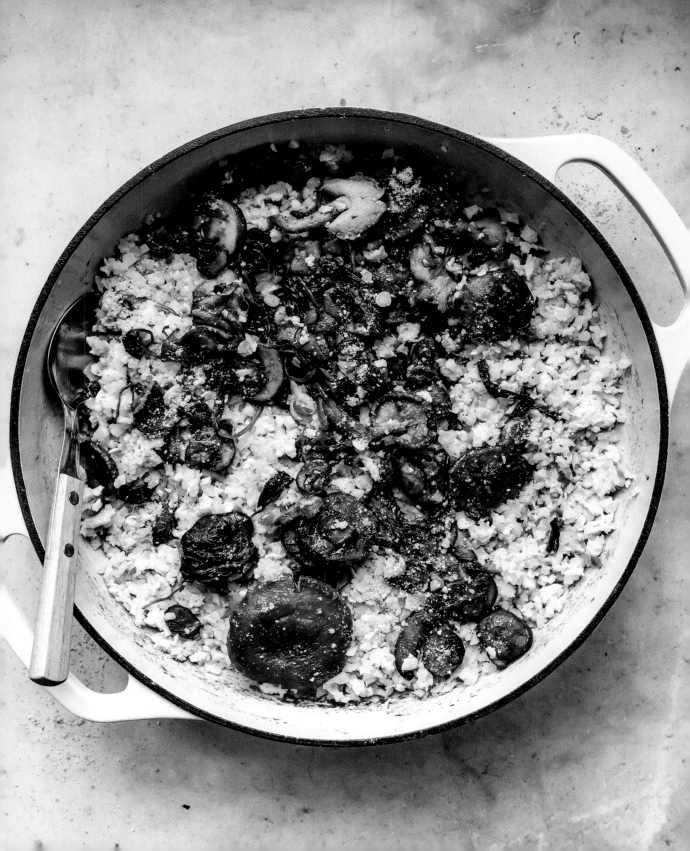

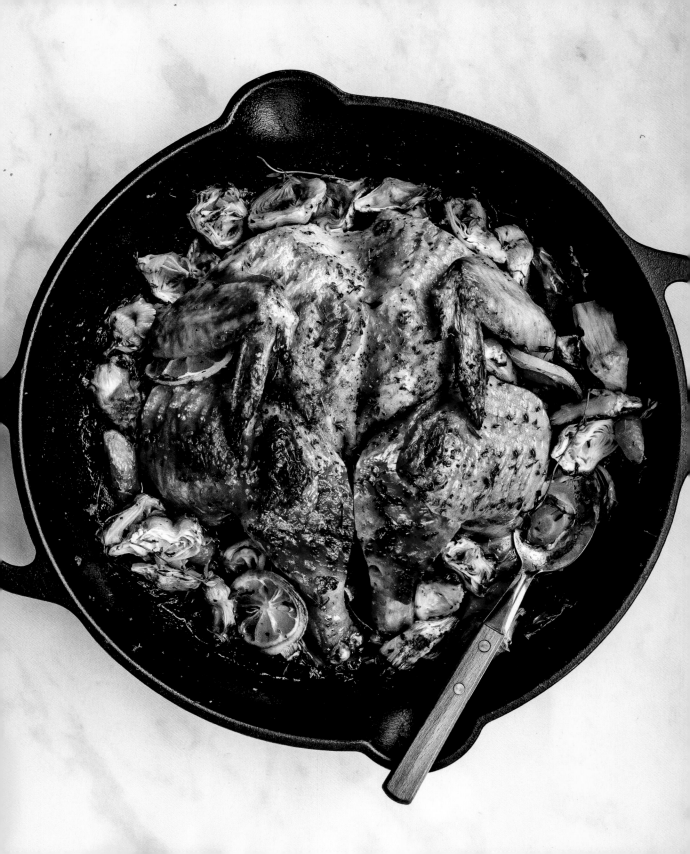

Lemon Spatchcock Chicken and Artichokes

Why spatchcock? Cutting open and flattening the chicken helps it to cook quicker and more evenly, with crispy skin and juicy meat. The pan sauce and veggies are caramelized and finger-licking good in this dish! Artichokes are high in fiber, and the bay leaves in the pan sauce help to alleviate gas, so I often use them in heavy vegetable dishes.

PREP TIME 10 minutes
COOK TIME 55 minutes
TOTAL TIME 1 hour and 5 minutes
YIELD 4 servings

1 whole (3–3½ lb., or 1.4–1.6 kg) organic, pasture-raised chicken

3–4 sprigs of thyme, plus more for garnish

3 tablespoons (45 ml) extra-virgin olive oil, divided

1 teaspoon sea salt, divided

¼ teaspoon black pepper (omit for AIP)

4 carrots, chopped

2 rutabagas or turnips, peeled and chopped

12 ounces (340 g) frozen and rinsed artichoke hearts

3 lemons (2 juiced and 1 sliced and zested)

To spatchcock the chicken: Pat your cleaned chicken dry and place on a cutting board, breast-side down, with the legs closest to you. Using kitchen shears or a sharp chef's knife, cut along one side of the spine. You can remove the spine for presentation purposes, but it's less effort to cook it along with your chicken and it will make a delicious broth later on! If you do remove the spine, I recommend baking it alongside your bird on a baking sheet to save for broth. Ensure you've cut all the way through the back and with both hands, pry the bird open so you can see the ribs and insides. Using a sharp knife, make a crack in the breast plate to help flatten the bird. Turn the bird over and firmly press the breasts down so the chicken can lay flat (or closer to it).

Add the bird to the center of a large cast-iron skillet or parchment paper-lined roasting pan, breast-side up. Tuck the sprigs of thyme into cavities with minimal exposure (They'll burn). Drizzle 1 tablespoon (15 ml) of oil over the bird, and sprinkle with ½ teaspoon of salt and pepper. Let the chicken sit and clean your hands.

Preheat the oven to 425°F (220°C, or gas mark 7) and arrange a rack in the middle.

In a mixing bowl, toss the veggies with remaining oil, lemon zest from 1 lemon, lemon juice of 2 lemons, and ½ teaspoon salt.

Add all veggies around the chicken and pour the juices in your pan (not over chicken). Place the pan in the oven and roast for 45 minutes. Rotate pan once halfway through, toss the vegetables, and add the lemon slices throughout the pan.

Prick the meat with a meat thermometer at the thickest part of the breast and thigh (not touching a bone). Be sure it reads 165°F (74°C). Remove from the oven and let rest uncovered for at least 10 minutes. Garnish with more thyme and lemon.

Crispy Golden Salmon

My now-husband and I used to make this dish in his tiny apartment kitchen in Queens, New York—usually setting off smoke alarms as we learned how to cook healthier together. To this day, we make this recipe constantly, switching it up, and we've come quite a long way confidence-wise since then! We love serving this alongside Rosemary Parsnip Puree (page 137) or Veggie Confetti Rice (page 133) with a green salad.

PREP TIME 5 minutes
COOK TIME 10 minutes
TOTAL TIME 15 minutes
YIELD 4 servings

RUB
¼ teaspoon sea salt

¼ teaspoon black pepper (omit for AIP)

½ teaspoon garlic powder

¼ teaspoon ground cinnamon

¼ teaspoon yellow curry powder (sub cinnamon for AIP)

¼ teaspoon ground cumin (sub ground ginger for AIP)

¼ teaspoon ground turmeric

SALMON
4 fillets (6 ounces, or 170 g) wild-caught salmon

1 tablespoon (15 ml) extra-virgin olive oil, divided

To make the rub: Combine all spices in a small mixing bowl.

To make the salmon: Pat the salmon dry on all sides and place it skin-side down on a cutting board. Brush 1 teaspoon of oil total across all salmon fillets and sprinkle the rub over each piece evenly. Rub the mixture in with your hands to coat.

Heat a cast-iron skillet or grill pan over medium heat and pour in remaining oil. Once the oil is shimmering, add salmon fillets flesh side (or seasoned side) down to the pan to sear. Let cook for 3 to 4 minutes before flipping it over to the skin side (or if no skin, just the other side) to cook for 5 to 6 minutes. For more well-done fish, you can cook it for an additional 2 to 3 minutes.

Using tongs or a spatula, wiggle salmon loose, and serve. If the skin is stuck, you can leave it alone to continue cooking for a few minutes until it comes loose.

Recipe Tip

Eat the skin! The highest concentration of omega-3s are in the skin. Just clean your fish before cooking it. The tastiest way to enjoy it is by grilling or pan-searing the fish as with this recipe so it's crisp (but not burned or smoking).

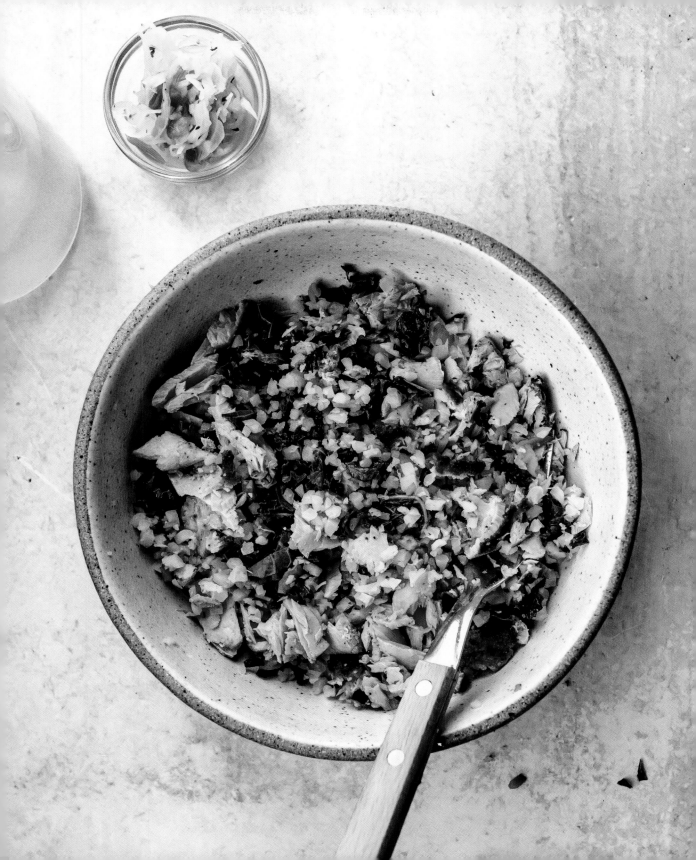

Meat Hash with Kale and Cabbage

I always have at least one batch of this easy meat hash in my fridge for breakfasts and lunches all week long. Mix up the meats, veggies, and seasonings, and use it as a base meal. I love it with a fried egg and avocado slices. It's an easy, nourishing breakfast and gives me the energy I need to run around after a toddler! Try it in a soup with bone broth, or stuffed inside a baked sweet potato with a little chimichurri sauce (page 191). Serve with a forkful of Fermented Coleslaw (page 184) to soothe your tummy and provide a dose of probiotics to the meal.

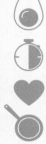

PREP TIME 8 minutes
COOK TIME 12 minutes
TOTAL TIME 20 minutes
YIELD 4 servings

1 tablespoon (15 ml) extra-virgin olive oil

1 pound (454 g) ground meat (such as organic pasture-raised poultry or grass-fed beef or bison)

1 tablespoon (3 g) dried rosemary, crushed

1 teaspoon sea salt, divided

2 cups (134 g) organic lacinato (or dino) kale, de-stemmed and chopped

2 cups (180 g) chopped purple cabbage

Heat a large sauté pan and add olive oil over medium heat. Add your meat and break it up with a wooden spoon as it cooks. Season with rosemary and ½ teaspoon salt.

Cook well for 10 minutes, or until you don't see any more raw meat. Add the veggies, stir, and cover for 3 to 5 minutes, until the veggies are soft and wilted. Season with ½ teaspoon of salt.

Herb-Stuffed Frittata

This frittata has so much amazing herby flavor, and of course the torn prosciutto on top gives it a crisp and salty layer of goodness. We love making this on the weekend to enjoy and have a few slices as leftover breakfasts for the week! Frittatas are a great way to use veggie leftovers; chop them up finely and toss in with the kale to precook before pouring in your eggs.

PREP TIME 5 minutes
COOK TIME 15 minutes
TOTAL TIME 20 minutes
YIELD 4 servings

8 pasture-raised eggs

¼ teaspoon sea salt

⅛ teaspoon black pepper

1½ tablespoons (4 g) chopped thyme

1 tablespoon (4 g) chopped oregano

1½ tablespoons (4 g) chopped chives

1½ tablespoons (5 g) chopped tarragon

2 tablespoons (30 ml) extra-virgin olive oil

1 cup (67 g) chopped baby kale

4 slices prosciutto, torn into pieces

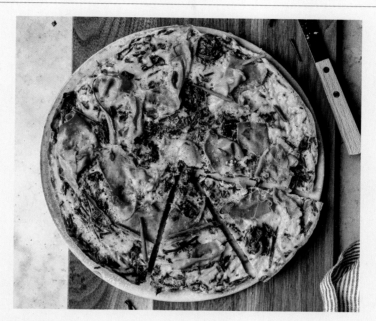

Preheat the oven to 400°F (200°C, or gas mark 6) and arrange a rack in the middle of the oven.

Beat eggs in a medium bowl with a whisk or fork until bubbles form. Season with salt, pepper, and all the herbs, beating them into the egg mixture until well combined.

Add the oil to a large oven-safe skillet (cast-iron works well) over medium heat. Add the kale for 2 minutes, stirring occasionally with a wooden spoon as it wilts. Pour the egg mixture in and tilt the pan to make sure the eggs settle evenly. Scatter the torn pieces of prosciutto evenly on top and cook for 1 to 2 minutes, until you see the eggs at the edges of the pan beginning to set.

Bake the frittata for 8 to 10 minutes, until the eggs are fully set in the middle. Carefully remove the skillet and let rest for a few minutes. Serve immediately, or store for up to 5 days in the fridge.

Recipe Tip

Skip this recipe on the elimination phase of AIP due to the eggs and choose the meat hash (page 94) instead.

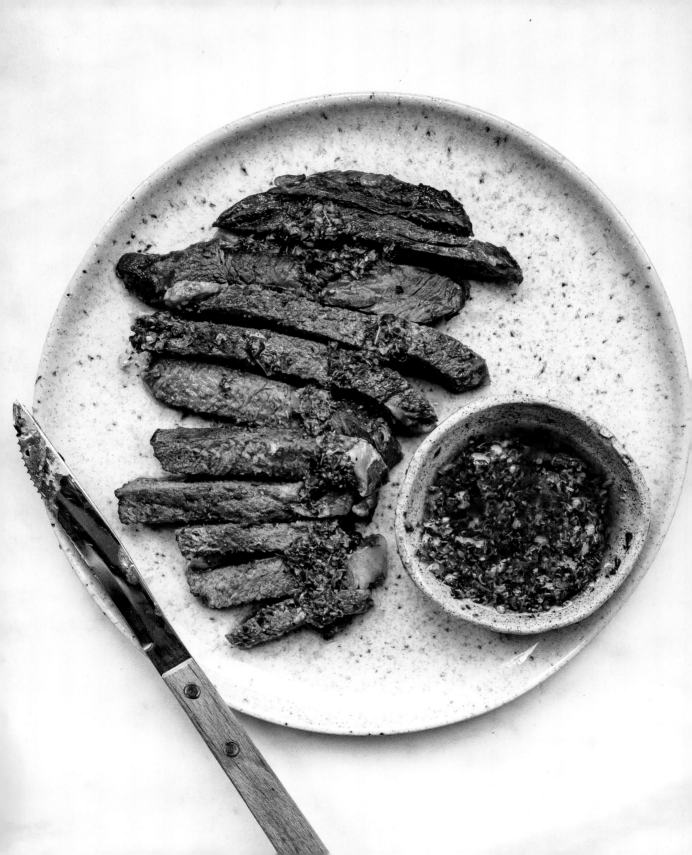

Rib Eye Steak with Chimichurri

Chimichurri elevates any dish, but especially a dish like this gorgeous rib eye steak! The garlicky-herby-tart goodness drizzled on a medium-cooked piece of meat is a match made in heaven. Serve this with Rosemary Parsnip Puree (page 137) or Crispy Baked Sweet Potato Fries (page 122) for a spin on the classic "steak and potatoes" dish.

PREP TIME 30 minutes
COOK TIME 15 minutes
TOTAL TIME 45 minutes
YIELD 4 servings

3–4 rib eye steaks (1 to 1½ inch thick, or 2.5 to 3.5 cm), preferably bone-in

2–3 tablespoons (28–45 ml) avocado oil, divided

1 tablespoon (18 g) sea salt

½ teaspoon black pepper (omit for AIP)

3–4 tablespoons (45–60 g) chimichurri sauce (page 191; modify for AIP)

Rinse and blot the steak dry with paper towels. Rub enough avocado oil to fully coat the steaks and season steaks on both sides with salt and pepper. Let sit at room temperature for 20 to 30 minutes. This isn't required, but helps the steak cook more evenly.

Heat the oven to 400°F (200°C, or gas mark 6).

On the stovetop, heat a large oven-safe or cast-iron skillet over medium-high heat until it's very hot.

Add the steaks, and carefully sear on each side for 2 minutes. Grab an oven mitt to carefully transfer the skillet into the oven to cook for 6 to 8 minutes depending on the desired doneness of the meat. (Remember they'll continue to cook outside of the oven, too.)

Take the steaks out and let them rest for 3 to 4 minutes while you plate and finish up sides. Serve the steak with or without the bone, and a drizzle of chimichurri.

"Cheesesteak" Stuffed Sweet Potatoes

If you have kids or picky eaters at home and are aching to get them eating your food, this would be a perfect gateway recipe. It's also a decadent comfort food for YOU. Add a forkful of sauerkraut, Fermented Coleslaw (page 184), or a dollop of Instant Pot Coconut Yogurt (page 187) to the top of your cheesesteak potatoes for a dose of probiotics and a boost of flavor!

PREP TIME 10 minutes
COOK TIME 45 minutes
TOTAL TIME 55 minutes
YIELD 4 servings

4 small sweet potatoes

1–2 tablespoons (15–30 ml) extra-virgin olive oil

2 pounds (907 g) rib eye, sirloin, or flank steak, sliced thinly

1 teaspoon sea salt, divided

¼ teaspoon black pepper (omit for AIP)

1 small yellow onion, sliced

½ cup (125 g) "cheese" sauce (page 188)

Chopped chives (optional)

Preheat the oven to 400°F (200°C, or gas mark 6) and arrange a rack on the lowest position of the oven. Line a baking sheet with parchment paper and set aside.

Poke the sweet potatoes a few times on all sides with a sharp knife and add them to the baking sheet. Roast for 40 minutes (depending on the thickness of potato), until cooked throughout.

To a skillet, heat 1 tablespoon (15 ml) of oil over medium heat and add the sliced steak and season with ½ teaspoon salt and pepper while sautéing for 3 to 4 minutes, until cooked. Set aside on a plate.

If needed, add 1 tablespoon (15 ml) of oil to the skillet and add the onions. Sauté and mix with a wooden spoon, until translucent and soft. Season with ½ teaspoon salt and remove from the heat. Add the onions to the plate of cooked meat and mix together.

Remove sweet potatoes from the oven (leave the heat on), and carefully slice them down the middle, lengthwise to open them up. Carefully squeeze the potatoes at each end to open them. With a fork, lightly mix up the middle sweet potato flesh and make some room for the filling. Using tongs or a large spoon, add the sliced steak and onions, packing it in evenly among potatoes.

Drizzle 1 to 2 tablespoons of "cheese" sauce on top and return the baking sheet to the oven to warm up the filling more for 5 to 10 minutes before serving. Garnish with chives (if using).

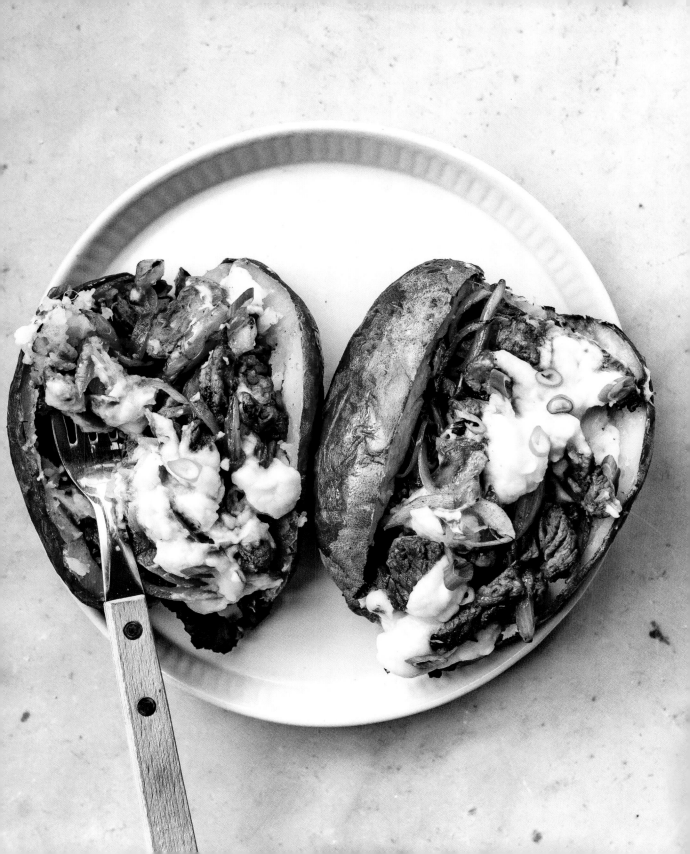

Crispy Roasted Chicken Thighs with Salsa Verde

A no-fuss, crispy chicken meal you can throw in the oven on any weeknight or dress up when entertaining! Have fun with different sauces here or go naked if you don't have any! They're delicious either way. If you're prepping these for leftovers, reheat them in the oven to get a nice crisp on the skin.

PREP TIME 5 minutes
COOK TIME 40 minutes
TOTAL TIME 45 minutes
YIELD 4 servings

2–3 pounds (907 g to 1.4 kg) bone-in chicken thighs, with skin

2 teaspoons sea salt

½ teaspoon black pepper (omit for AIP)

½ cup (120 g) salsa verde (page 192)

Preheat the oven to 400°F (200°C, or gas mark 6) and prepare a baking sheet with parchment paper with a grate on top so all parts will be crispy and evenly cooked.

Rinse the chicken thighs and pat them dry with a paper towel so the skin will be crispy.

Season chicken thighs with salt and pepper on both sides.

Place chicken thighs skin-side up on the grates and bake for 35 to 45 minutes. They're done when a meat thermometer reads 165°F (74°C) in the thickest part of the thigh (not touching the bone).

Serve your chicken with a side of salsa verde and your favorite sides.

Sweet-and-Sour Meatballs with Roasted Cauliflower

This is a Paleo-fied version of a delightful sheet pan recipe from *Bon Appétit* magazine. Inspired by Japanese grilled chicken meatballs (*tsukune*), this sweet-and-sour gingery dish is a savory dream. Use the sauce as an alternate on the Teriyaki Salmon and Bok Choy (page 102) or slathered on some grilled pork chops. Adding ginger to this sauce will help you break down the protein from the meatballs—plus it tastes fantastic!

PREP TIME 15 minutes
COOK TIME 20 minutes
TOTAL TIME 35 minutes
YIELD 4 servings

SWEET-AND-SOUR SAUCE

½ cup (120 g) ketchup (or AIP-compliant beet ketchup for AIP replacement)

3 tablespoons (45 ml) coconut aminos

2 tablespoons (28 ml) balsamic vinegar

2 tablespoons (40 g) raw honey

1 tablespoon (6 g) minced ginger or 1 teaspoon powder

MEATBALLS AND VEGGIES

4 cups (528 g) cauliflower florets

2 carrots, chopped into 1-inch (2.5-cm)-thick rounds

2 tablespoons (30 ml) avocado oil, divided

1½ teaspoons sea salt, divided

1 pound (454 g) free-range organic ground turkey or chicken

1 tablespoon (9 g) arrowroot

1 teaspoon garlic powder

2 teaspoons onion powder

¼ teaspoon black pepper (omit for AIP)

2 teaspoons toasted sesame oil (omit for AIP)

Finely chopped scallions and sesame seeds (optional; omit seeds for AIP)

To make the sweet-and-sour sauce: Combine all the ingredients in a small saucepan. Whisk while bringing to a simmer over medium heat for 4 to 5 minutes, until the sauce thickens and reduces. Remove from the heat and set aside.

To make the meatballs and veggies: Arrange racks in the middle of the oven and heat to 450°F (230°C, or gas mark 8). Line 2 baking sheets with parchment paper.

Add the cauliflower and carrots to one sheet in a single layer. Drizzle 1 tablespoon (15 ml) of avocado oil over veggies and season with 1 teaspoon salt, lightly tossing.

In a large mixing bowl, add the meat, arrowroot, garlic powder, onion powder, pepper, and ½ teaspoon salt together. Mix by hand until well combined. Form into meatballs (10 to 12 total using a tablespoon). Arrange the meatballs in a single layer on the second lined baking sheet.

Add the pans to the oven and bake for 15 minutes, until meatballs are cooked through. Remove from the oven and turn on the broiler. To your pan, brush or drizzle meatballs with half of the reserved sauce. Place meatballs under the broiler for 3 to 4 minutes until sauce is bubbling and veggies are browned and slightly charred in the oven. Remove both pans from the oven. To the remaining sauce, mix in the toasted sesame oil and drizzle the sauce over meatballs and veggies to taste before serving. Garnish with scallions and sesame seeds.

Teriyaki Salmon and Bok Choy

Sheet pan meals are such a favorite because it's no-fuss and less cleanup. Here's another perfect weeknight meal bursting with flavor for you to enjoy. Serve alongside simple sautéed cauliflower rice, if you'd like!

PREP TIME 5 minutes
COOK TIME 20 minutes
TOTAL TIME 25 minutes
YIELD 4 servings

TERIYAKI SAUCE
¼ cup (60 ml) coconut aminos

3 tablespoons (60 g) raw honey

1 teaspoon grated ginger or
¼ teaspoon powder

2 teaspoons arrowroot

2 cloves garlic, minced

1 tablespoon (15 ml) toasted
sesame oil (sub olive oil for AIP)

SALMON AND BOK CHOY
4 fillets (6 ounces, or 170 g)
wild-caught salmon

4 pieces baby bok choy,
halved lengthwise

1 tablespoon (15 ml) extra-virgin
olive oil

½ teaspoon sea salt

¼ teaspoon black pepper
(omit for AIP)

2 scallions, finely chopped

Sesame seeds (optional;
omit for AIP)

Preheat the oven to 425°F (220°C, or gas mark 7) and line a baking sheet with parchment paper.

To make the sauce: Combine all the ingredients, except toasted sesame oil, in a small saucepan. Whisk together and bring to a low simmer for 3 to 4 minutes, and then remove from the heat and mix in the toasted sesame oil. Set aside.

To make the salmon: Place salmon fillets and bok choy in a single layer on the lined baking sheet.

Spoon teriyaki sauce over the salmon (reserving half for later). Drizzle oil over the bok choy, and season with salt and pepper.

Place everything in the oven for 12 to 15 minutes, or until salmon is cooked and flakes with a fork and the bok choy is tender and lightly charred on top.

Plate the salmon and bok choy, drizzling with the reserved sauce and garnishing with the scallions and sesame seeds (if using).

Shrimp and Broccoli

I'm all about a 30-minute weeknight meal, and this easy recipe is fast and flavorful. Who needs takeout when you've got wholesome ingredients you can whip up some "fakeout" with at home?! Use this same recipe and sub the protein with thinly sliced chicken breast or beef. Just cook it a bit longer! It's interchangeable and so tasty.

PREP TIME 10 minutes
COOK TIME 20 minutes
TOTAL TIME 30 minutes
YIELD 4 servings

SHRIMP MARINADE

2 tablespoons (28 ml) coconut aminos

1 tablespoon (15 ml) olive oil

½ teaspoon ground ginger/juice or 1 teaspoon grated

1 tablespoon (7 g) garlic powder or 3 cloves garlic, minced

¼ teaspoon ground turmeric

¼ teaspoon fish sauce (optional)

SHEET PAN

2 pounds (907 g) frozen or fresh shrimp, peeled and deveined

12 ounces (340 g) broccoli florets

4 carrots, chopped into 1-inch (2.5-cm) pieces

1 tablespoon (15 ml) extra-virgin olive oil

½ teaspoon ground turmeric

½ teaspoon ground ginger

½ teaspoon garlic powder

¼ teaspoon sea salt

¼ teaspoon black pepper (omit for AIP)

1 teaspoon toasted sesame oil (omit for AIP)

Toasted sesame seeds (optional; omit for AIP)

¼ cup chopped scallions (optional)

Prepared cauliflower rice (optional)

Preheat the oven to 400°F (200°C, or gas mark 6), arrange a rack in the middle of the oven, and line a baking sheet with parchment paper.

To make the marinade: Assemble all the ingredients in a medium mixing bowl. Divide the marinade in half. Put half in a large mixing bowl and add your thawed/semi-thawed shrimp to marinate. Set the remaining marinade aside to use as a finishing sauce.

To make the sheet pan: Add the broccoli and carrots to the sheet pan in a single layer, allowing some room to place the shrimp later. Drizzle with oil, turmeric, ginger, garlic powder, salt, and pepper. Toss to coat.

Roast for 10 minutes. Remove the sheet pan from the oven, nudge veggies to the side, and place your marinated shrimp on the free side. Be careful to not let too much excess marinade onto the pan. Roast for 10 to 12 minutes, until the shrimp is tender and pink and the veggies are golden brown.

Drizzle with the reserved sauce and toasted sesame oil. Garnish with chopped scallions or toasted sesame seeds (if using). You can also serve this over some cauliflower rice if you'd like.

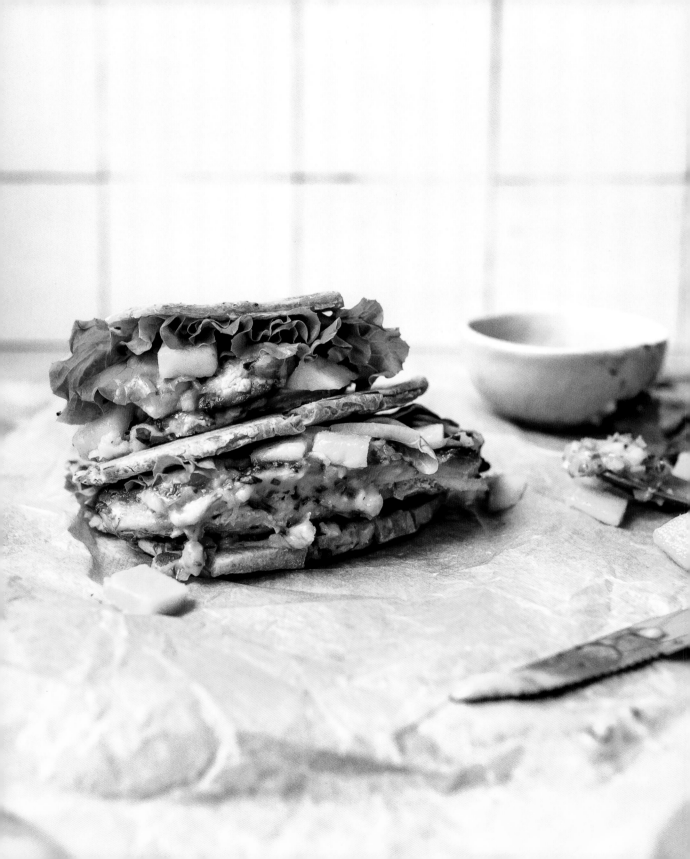

Mango Chicken Jibaritos *(Plantain Sandwiches)*

If you can name me a more versatile veggie than the plantain, you win some kind of award. Here, it is used as the bread for this refreshing mango chicken sandwich, and it couldn't be easier or tastier to make!

PREP TIME 10 minutes
COOK TIME 35 minutes
TOTAL TIME 45 minutes
YIELD 4 servings

PLANTAIN SANDWICH BREAD
2 green plantains

1 tablespoon (15 ml) extra-virgin olive oil

¼ teaspoon sea salt

SANDWICH FILLING
2 chicken breasts (1 pound, or 454 g), butterflied into 4 pieces or 4 chicken "cutlets"

½ teaspoon sea salt, divided

¼ teaspoon black pepper (omit for AIP)

4 teaspoons (20 ml) extra-virgin olive oil, divided

1 avocado, pitted and peeled

¼ cup (4 g) chopped cilantro

1 teaspoon lime juice

4 pieces romaine lettuce

¼ cup (65 g) mango salsa (page 193)

Preheat the oven to 350°F (175°C, or gas mark 4). Loosely line a baking sheet with tin foil; you'll need to pick up the tin foil midway. Have a second piece of tin foil or parchment paper ready.

To make the sandwich bread: Cut the plantains in the middle in half and peel off the skin. Cut each slice in half lengthwise so you have 4 pieces. Drizzle the baking sheet with oil and roll each plantain piece to coat them in the oil. Lay each on the flat sides and sprinkle with salt. Bake for 20 minutes. Keep the oven on, take out your pan, and move the tin foil and plantains to a cutting board. Lay the second piece of tin foil on top of the hot plantains and press each with a heavy pan to flatten. Flip each one and press again until you're happy with the size and thickness. If it cracks a little, it's okay—you can mend it together. Return the tin foil with plantains back to the baking sheet and bake for 10 minutes. Set aside.

To make the filling: Season the chicken with ¼ teaspoon salt and pepper and rub it with 2 teaspoons of oil on all sides. In a cast-iron skillet over medium heat, add 2 teaspoons of oil. Once shimmering, add the chicken pieces and cook on each side for 3 to 4 minutes, until cooked through. It should be 165°F (74°C). Set the chicken aside to rest without cutting so it stays moist.

To a food processor, add the avocado, cilantro, lime juice, and ¼ teaspoon salt. Pulse until you have a spread consistency. Taste and adjust seasonings and lime juice, if needed.

Spread cilantro-lime sauce on your bottom sandwich plantain slices. Add a slice of romaine and a chicken piece, and top with salsa and your top piece of plantain. To make these ahead, store everything separately, reheat the plantains, and assemble.

Pastelón (*Puerto Rican Casserole*)

I grew up making this dish with my mom, grandmother, and great-aunts while telling stories and laughing in Spanglish. Every family does theirs differently; mine puts raisins and olives in the picadillo. Here, I'm making it with plantains and mashed cauliflower, and it's *delicioso*!

PREP TIME 30 minutes
COOK TIME 1 hour
TOTAL TIME 1 hour and 30 minutes
YIELD 6 to 8 servings

PICADILLO
2 medium yellow onions, finely chopped

3 tablespoons (45 ml) extra-virgin olive oil

4 cloves garlic, minced

2 pounds (907 g) ground beef or bison

½ teaspoon sea salt

¼ teaspoon black pepper (omit for AIP)

1 tablespoon (3 g) dried oregano

2 teaspoons ground cumin (sub cinnamon for AIP)

⅓ cup (5 g) chopped cilantro, plus more for garnish

3–4 tablespoons (48–64 g) tomato paste (omit for AIP)

½ cup (120 ml) basic broth or bone, store-bought or homemade (page 182 or 183)

½ cup (50 g) chopped green pitted olives

⅓ cup (50 g) raisins

MASHED CAULIFLOWER
2 cups (475 ml) water

2 pounds (907 g) cauliflower florets

2 tablespoons (30 ml) extra-virgin olive oil

½ teaspoon sea salt

SWEET PLANTAINS
1 teaspoon extra-virgin olive oil

3–4 ripe plantains (yellow)

½ teaspoon sea salt

To make the picadillo: Over medium heat, sauté the onion in the oil for 8 to 10 minutes, until soft and translucent. Add the garlic and stir with a wooden spoon for 30 seconds and add the ground meat, breaking up with a wooden spoon. Season with salt and pepper. Add the oregano, cumin, and cilantro. Keep breaking up the meat and cook for 5 minutes, until most of the pink is gone. Stir in the tomato paste and broth, and mix very well. Simmer for 10 minutes, stirring occasionally. Add your olives and raisins. Simmer for 10 minutes, then adjust any seasonings as you'd like! Set aside.

To make the cauliflower: Bring the water to a boil and add the cauliflower to a steam basket. Cover and cook for 5 to 7 minutes, until fork-tender. Remove the florets and add to a food processor, in batches if needed. Pulse until mashed, then spoon out into a large bowl. Alternatively, mash with a potato masher in a large bowl. Add the oil and season with salt, mixing as you season. Set aside.

To assemble: Preheat the oven to 350°F (175°C, or gas mark 4) and place a shelf in the middle. Grease a 13 x 9-inch (33 x 23-cm) baking dish with 1 teaspoon of oil

Chop off ends of the plantains, cut widthwise, and score the skin so you can peel it off. Carefully slice the plantains into thin slices lengthwise; I usually get 4 to 5 slices from each half.

Press in half your mashed cauliflower in an even layer in the baking dish. Add a layer of picadillo, followed by a layer of raw plantains. The plantains will shrink; it's okay to overlap a bit. Do one more round of layers and sprinkle a ½ teaspoon of salt.

Place baking dish on a baking sheet and cover the baking dish with foil or an oven-safe top. Bake for 1 hour. Remove from the oven and let sit for 5-10 minutes before slicing and serving. This will keep for up to 6 days in an airtight container.

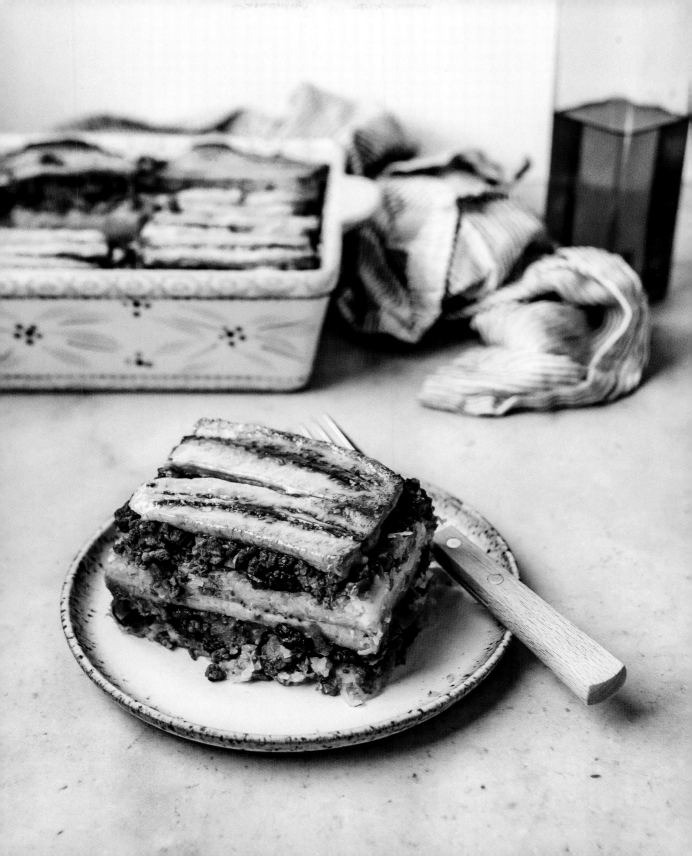

Spaghetti Squash Pastitsio *(Greek Baked Ziti)*

My husband exposed me to pastitsio on a date in Astoria, New York City. It was like opening Pandora's box! I've re-created its magic using spaghetti squash in place of pasta and a dairy-free sauce with béchamel-like consistency. It's easy on the tummy and a treat for the taste buds.

PREP TIME 15 minutes

COOK TIME 1 hour and 30 minutes

TOTAL TIME 1 hour and 45 minutes

YIELD 4 to 6 servings

SPAGHETTI SQUASH LAYER

2 medium spaghetti squash (4–5 cups, or 1 kg–1.3 kg cooked)

1 tablespoon (15 ml) extra-virgin olive oil

GROUND MEAT LAYER

2 tablespoons (30 ml) extra-virgin olive oil

1 small yellow onion, chopped

1 pound (454 g) grass-fed ground beef or lamb

2 teaspoons dried oregano

1 teaspoon sea salt

2 teaspoons ground cinnamon

2 teaspoons tomato paste (omit for AIP)

3 cloves garlic, minced

DAIRY-FREE CAULIFLOWER BÉCHAMEL SAUCE

1 batch "cheese" sauce (page 188)

¼ cup (60 ml) water, if needed

NUTRITIONAL YEAST-CINNAMON TOPPING

2 tablespoons (10 g) nutritional yeast flakes

1–2 teaspoons ground cinnamon

1 pinch sea salt

To make the squash: Preheat the oven to 400°F (200°C, or gas mark 6). Line a baking sheet with parchment paper. Cut the squash into 1-inch (2.5-cm) rings and discard seeds. Drizzle oil on both sides of the rings and bake on the baking sheet for 30 minutes, flipping halfway. Set aside.

Reduce the oven temperature to 350°F (175°C, or gas mark 4) and grease an 8 x 8–inch (20 x 20–cm) baking dish. Set aside.

To make the meat: In a skillet over medium heat, add the oil. Once shimmering, add the onions and stir using a wooden spoon for 3 to 5 minutes, until translucent and soft. Add the meat and break it up. Add the seasonings, tomato paste, and garlic and cook for 3 to 4 minutes more, until the juices start to evaporate and no red remains. Set aside.

To assemble: In a bowl, combine the "cheese" sauce with water if needed to loosen it. Set aside. To your baking dish, add two-thirds of your spaghetti squash and pack it in a single layer with a fork (no empty pockets). Add in the meat, packing it in well with a fork in a single layer. Pour two-thirds of the sauce over. Use a wooden spoon to push the sauce to cover the meat fully. If the sauce covered the meat well, you're in good shape. If more liquid is needed, add that to the remaining sauce in the blender and blend it on high for 30 seconds.

With your hands, pull apart the remaining one-third of squash to the width of your baking dish. Place the squash "in stripes" so that it's an even, single layer but not sinking into the sauce. Add the remaining sauce, pushing with your wooden spoon to cover the squash. Add your topping lightly and evenly over the dish.

Bake for 40 minutes, until the top is golden brown and bubbling on the edges. Let rest for 5 to 10 minutes before cutting. This will keep well in the fridge for 1 week.

Moussaka *(Greek Eggplant Casserole)*

Layers of delish eggplant, lamb, and a dairy-free béchamel make a comforting casserole that is perfect for a hearty Sunday meal or batching for meal prep! You can also substitute beef or bison for the lamb.

PREP TIME 30 minutes

COOK TIME 1 hour and 10 minutes

TOTAL TIME 1 hour and 40 minutes

YIELD 6 to 8 servings

1 medium eggplant, sliced crosswise into ¼-inch (6-mm)-thick rounds

¼ cup (59 ml) plus 2 tablespoons (30 ml) extra-virgin olive oil, divided

1 teaspoon sea salt, divided

1 tablespoon (3 g) dried oregano

1 pound (454 g) ground lamb or other ground meat

1 teaspoon paprika

2 teaspoons ground cinnamon

1 medium onion, chopped

1 tablespoon (6 g) chopped mint, divided

4 cloves garlic, finely grated, divided

1 tablespoon (16 g) tomato paste

¼ cup (60 ml) bone broth, store-bought or homemade (page 183)

2–3 vine tomatoes, peeled and chopped

1 batch of "cheese" sauce (page 188)

Preheat the oven to 400°F (200°C, or gas mark 6) and place a rack in the middle. Line a large baking sheet with parchment paper.

Coat the eggplant with ¼ cup (59 ml) of oil, and add it to the baking sheet. Season with ½ teaspoon of salt and the oregano. Bake in a single layer and roast for 30 minutes, until cooked and golden, flipping after 15 minutes.

Meanwhile, add 2 tablespoons (30 ml) of oil to a large skillet over medium heat. Add the lamb, remaining salt, paprika, and cinnamon. Cook and break up with a wooden spoon for 10 minutes, until browned on all sides and liquid from the meat is evaporating. Remove the meat from the pan and set aside, leaving fat in the pan (or adding more if needed).

Add the onion and mint, and season with remaining ½ teaspoon of salt. Sauté for 5 to 8 minutes, until translucent. Add garlic for 1 to 2 minutes. Add the tomato paste, stir, and add your broth. Cook for 3 minutes, stirring occasionally.

Add the tomatoes and the lamb. Cook for 5 to 7 minutes, stirring occasionally, until most of the liquid is evaporated and mixture looks like a thick meat sauce.

To assemble: Grease an 8 x 8–inch (20 x 20–cm) baking pan with oil. Layer half of the eggplant in the pan, covering the bottom. Evenly spread half of the lamb mixture over the eggplant. Repeat with remaining eggplant and lamb to make another layer of each. Top with sauce and smooth the surface. Bake the moussaka for 30 to 45 minutes, until bubbling and browned in spots. Let cool 5 to 10 minutes before serving.

Recipe Tip

In the elimination phase of AIP, skip this dish and try the Spaghetti Squash Pastitsio on the opposite page, which is a perfect swap!

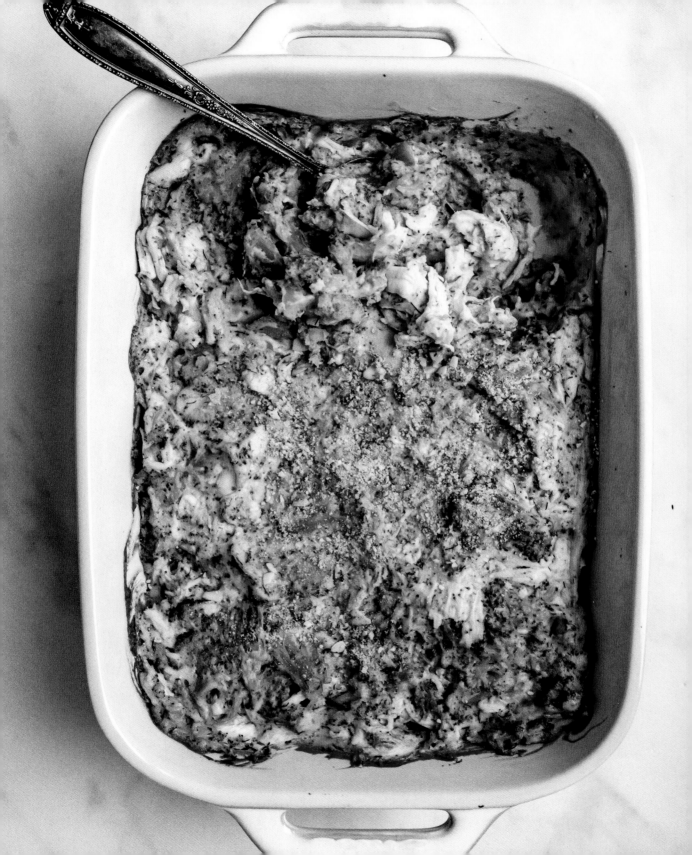

Creamy Chicken and Broccoli Bake

I remember the days when my mom would make a delicious cheesy casserole because anything covered in cheese would please us kids and my dad! Especially if broccoli was involved. This is an ode to late nights working with my parents on homework after their long days of work. Here's to one-pot cheesy surprises, minus the cheese! This is great for meal prep or on any weeknight.

PREP TIME 10 minutes
COOK TIME 25 minutes
TOTAL TIME 35 minutes
YIELD 4 servings

3 cups (705 ml) filtered water

4 cups (284 g) broccoli florets

1 batch "cheese" sauce (page 188)

¼ cup (60 g) unsweetened coconut yogurt, optional (homemade, page 187, or additive-free if store-bought)

1 teaspoon garlic powder

1 teaspoon onion powder

½ teaspoon ground turmeric

½ teaspoon dried dill

1 teaspoon sea salt

¼ teaspoon black pepper (omit for AIP)

4 cups (560 g) or 2 skinless cooked chicken breasts, shredded (page 74)

Pepitasan (optional, omit for AIP; page 88)

Preheat the oven to 375°F (190°C, or gas mark 5) and place a rack in the middle. Bring a large pot of water to boil. Add the broccoli and cook for 3 minutes. Remove from the heat and drain. Set aside.

In a medium mixing bowl, add the cheese sauce, coconut yogurt (if using), and all the seasonings.

To an 8- to 10-inch (20- to 25-cm) baking dish or cast-iron skillet, add the chicken and broccoli, pour the cheese sauce mixture, and stir with a spatula. Bake for 20 minutes, until the cheese sauce is browning on the edges. Remove from the oven. Sprinkle with pepitasan topping (if using), and serve alone or with a side salad.

Greek Stuffed Cabbage Rolls in Lemony Sauce

Once you make cabbage rolls, you'll wonder why you hadn't before. Here we are making a spin on a classic Greek dish called *Lahanodolmades*. It's similar to stuffed grape leaves (*dolmades*)!

PREP TIME 15 minutes
COOK TIME 1 hour
TOTAL TIME 1 hour and 15 minutes
YIELD 4 servings

LEMON CREAM SAUCE
1 white sweet potato, peeled and diced
1 cup (235 ml) filtered water
½ cup (120 ml) fresh lemon juice

CABBAGE AND FILLING
1 head of cabbage, stem removed
1 pound (454 g) grass-fed ground beef, bison, or lamb
1 small yellow onion, chopped
½ teaspoon sea salt
¼ teaspoon black pepper (omit for AIP)
⅓ cup (20 g) chopped parsley
⅓ cup (21 g) chopped dill
1 tablespoon (15 ml) extra-virgin olive oil
Cauliflower rice (optional)

Add the sweet potato to a pot along with enough water to cover. Boil for 10 to 12 minutes, until fork-tender. Drain and add the potatoes to a blender with the water and juice to form a puree.

In a large, heavy-bottomed pot, bring to boil enough water to cover the whole cabbage (don't add it yet). Cover and let the water boil while you make the filling.

Mix the meat, onion, salt, pepper, and herbs together in a mixing bowl by hand until well combined. Fill a large bowl with ice cubes and cold water, set aside.

Using tongs, lower the cabbage into the boiling water. Boil for 1 to 2 minutes. Remove carefully and place it in a large bowl. Peel back the soft leaves, placing each in the ice water.

Preheat your oven to 350°F (175°C, or gas mark 4). Grease a large baking dish with the oil. Pat each leaf dry and lay them on a cutting board with the core-side facing you. Snip any hard pieces from the remaining core in ½ to 1 inch (1.3 to 2.5 cm) in a "v" pattern to make it easier to roll.

Separate the meat mixture to create as many pieces as you have leaves. (If you have 10 good leaves, score the meat 10 ways.) Spoon 1 to 2 heaping tablespoons of mixture onto the bottom of the leaf. Fold the sides in, and then fold the bottom away from you to the top of the leaf. Keep the edge tucked underneath.

Add the rolls in a single layer, packed next to one another. Pile them on top or squeeze them in so they don't come undone. Pour the sauce on top and give the dish a shake to coat.

Cover the dish with parchment paper and then aluminum foil on top tightly. Bake for 1 hour, or until cooked through and the cabbage is tender. Serve with sauce over cauliflower rice (if using).

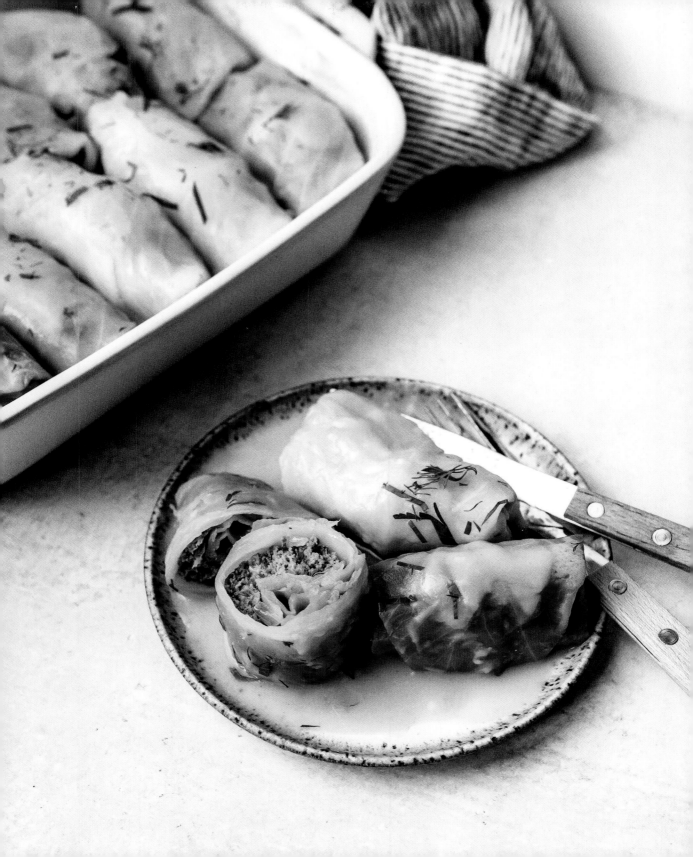

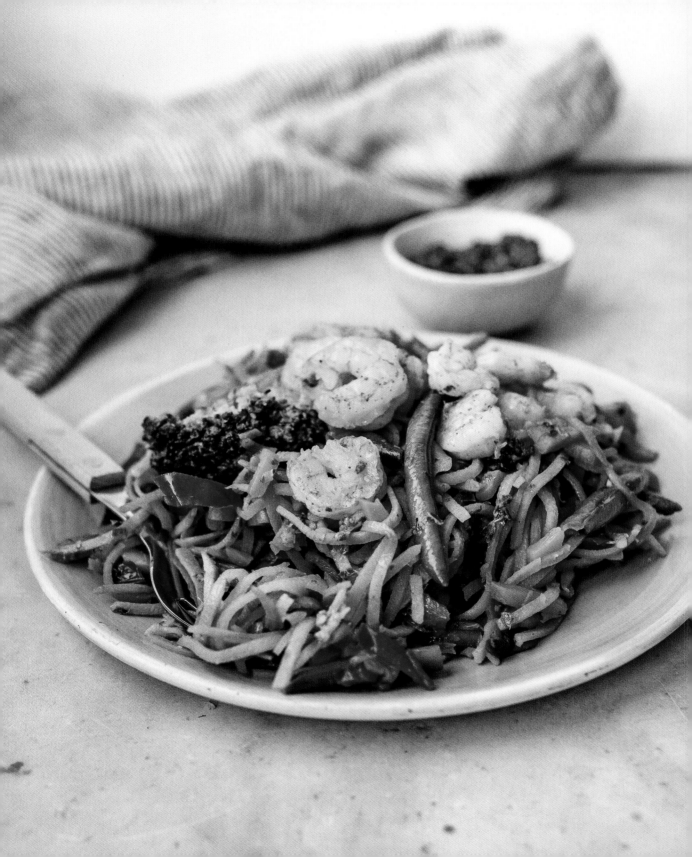

Pesto Primavera Veggie Noodles with Shrimp

When I embarked on my healthy eating journey, veggie noodles from zucchini ("zoodles") and butternut squash (or "boodles", as I call them) were a fun way to re-create my favorite pasta dishes. This dish is packed with vegetables and garlicky pesto for a true "pasta primavera." Choose broccoli, cauliflower, carrots, mushrooms, or asparagus and make it AIP-friendly. Swap the shrimp for scallops, salmon, or shredded chicken (page 74). Try a forkful of Fermented Coleslaw (page 184) or a dollop of tangy Instant Pot Coconut Yogurt (page 187) in place of traditional cheese or stir it in for a creamier dish!

PREP TIME 10 minutes
COOK TIME 20 minutes
TOTAL TIME 30 minutes
YIELD 4 to 6 servings

KALE PESTO
4 cups (268 g) de-stemmed and ripped kale

½ cup (20 g) basil leaves

2 cloves garlic, minced

2 teaspoons nutritional yeast

⅓ cup (79 ml) extra-virgin olive oil, plus more if needed

½ teaspoon sea salt, plus more to taste

¼ teaspoon black pepper (omit for AIP)

1 teaspoon fresh lemon juice

VEGGIE NOODLES AND SHRIMP
2 pounds (907 g) frozen or fresh shrimp, peeled and deveined

3 tablespoons (45 ml) extra-virgin olive oil, divided

1½ teaspoons sea salt, divided

½ teaspoon black pepper (omit for AIP), divided

Zest from 1 lemon

2 rutabagas, peeled and spiralized

16 ounces (455 g) frozen vegetable mix or 2 cups (260 g) chopped vegetables

To make the pesto: Mix all the ingredients in a food processor and set aside.

To make the noodles and shrimp: In a mixing bowl, toss the thawed shrimp in 1 tablespoon (15 ml) of oil and season with ½ teaspoon salt, ¼ teaspoon pepper, and lemon zest.

To a cast-iron or large skillet over medium heat, add 2 tablespoons (30 ml) of oil. Once shimmering, add the shrimp and cook on each side for 1 to 2 minutes, until pink and tender. Transfer the shrimp to a plate using tongs and set aside, reserving the oil in the skillet.

To the skillet, add the rutabaga noodles, tossing in the oil for 2 to 3 minutes over medium heat. Add the vegetables and salt. Continue cooking for 7 to 10 minutes, mixing occasionally, until all vegetables are fork-tender.

Pour in 2 tablespoons (30 g) of pesto and mix with tongs to coat your noodles and veggies. Add more pesto to taste. If the pesto is thick, you can loosen it with a little more oil. Top with shrimp, remove from the heat, and serve. Squeeze remaining lemon juice over the top, if you'd like.

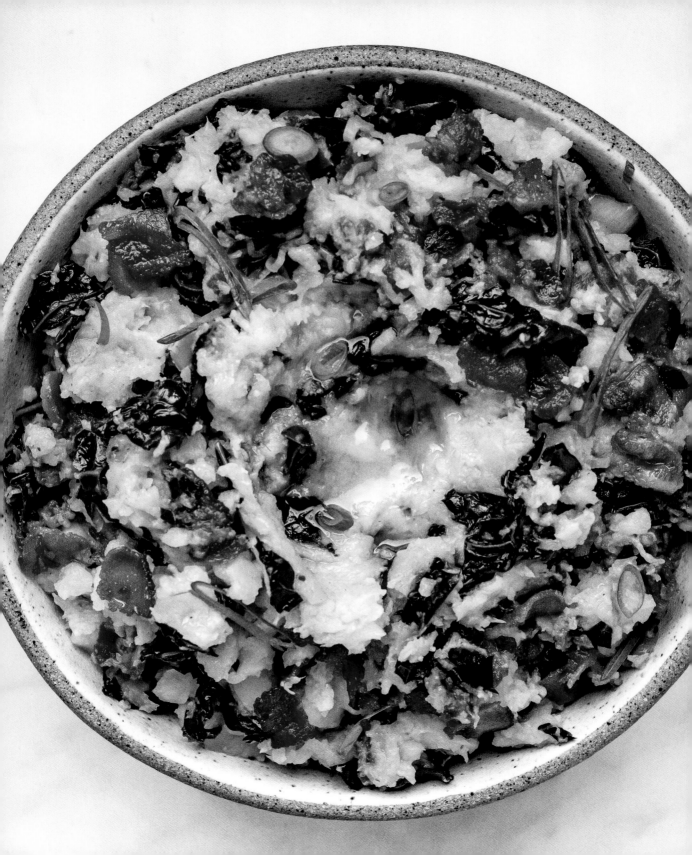

5

VEGGIES
& SIDES

Loading your plate with veggies is part of the game here in Paleo-land! Simple tossed greens, sautéed cauliflower rice, and roasted vegetables are easy sides to any dish. And I've got more ideas for you in this section to keep it fresh. Substitute vegetables based on your taste, what's in season, or what's available. Have fun with it!

———————————

Tostones with Mango Salsa *(Fried Green Plantains)* 118

Bone Broth Garlic Kale 121

Crispy Baked Sweet Potato Fries 122

Creamy Mashed Cauliflower with Mushroom Gravy 125

Irish Colcannon 126

Fasolakia *(Haricots Verts in Tomato Sauce)* 129

Bone Broth Mangú with Salsa Verde 130

Veggie Confetti Rice 133

Ginger Balsamic Beets and Greens 134

Rosemary Parsnip Puree 137

Tostones with Mango Salsa
(Fried Green Plantains)

Growing up, fried plantains were my favorite. I have loving memories of my grandparents frying them up—sweet (*maduros*) or salty (*tostones*)—while I devoured them before they made it to the table! They make a great side or "cracker." I've paired them with delicious mango salsa.

PREP TIME 10 minutes
COOK TIME 20 minutes
TOTAL TIME 30 minutes
YIELD 4 servings

2–3 very green unripe plantains

4 cups (940 ml) filtered water

1 teaspoon sea salt, divided

1½ teaspoons onion powder

1½ teaspoons garlic powder

½ cup (109 g) animal fat such as tallow or lard, coconut oil, or avocado oil for frying (Have more handy in case you need more.)

1 batch mango salsa (page 193)

Lime and cilantro (optional)

Chop the ends off the plantains and score the peel with a knife down the center, lengthwise. Peel them and chop into 1-inch (2.5-cm) sections.

Place the water, ½ teaspoon salt, onion powder, and garlic powder in a large baking dish and place near the stove.

If you have a "tostonera" press, place a piece of parchment paper to cover the top and bottom of it inside. Alternatively, simply put a piece of the parchment paper on a cutting board. Have a skillet or plate nearby; you'll use it to flatten the plantains (using a second sheet of parchment paper so it doesn't stick).

Heat a large skillet over medium-high heat and add your fat. Once the fat is shimmering, check that it's 365°F (185°C). Or place a wooden spoon in the oil and if it crackles, it's ready. Add the plantains and fry on both sides, until golden-yellow on each side, flipping with tongs.

Transfer the pieces to your pressing station and press your plantains between the sheets of parchment paper. Press firmly but not excessively, until they're ¼ inch (6 mm) thick. Once you press, place each one in the seasoned water to sit for a couple of minutes while you continue pressing the plantains. This step makes for a soft center with a crispy exterior!

Using tongs, lift the plantains out of the water and shake off excess water. Then dip it on a paper towel and place it back into the oil. You may need to do this in batches this time because fewer will fit in the oil. Continue cooking, until crispy and golden brown.

Remove each toston from the oil when done and sprinkle with more salt to taste. Serve immediately with your prepared mango salsa and garnish with some lime and cilantro (if using).

Recipe Tip

These are best served and eaten right away. Shortcut: If you don't want to dip in the seasoned water, you can season them with onion and garlic powder after pressing them flat and before frying the second time!

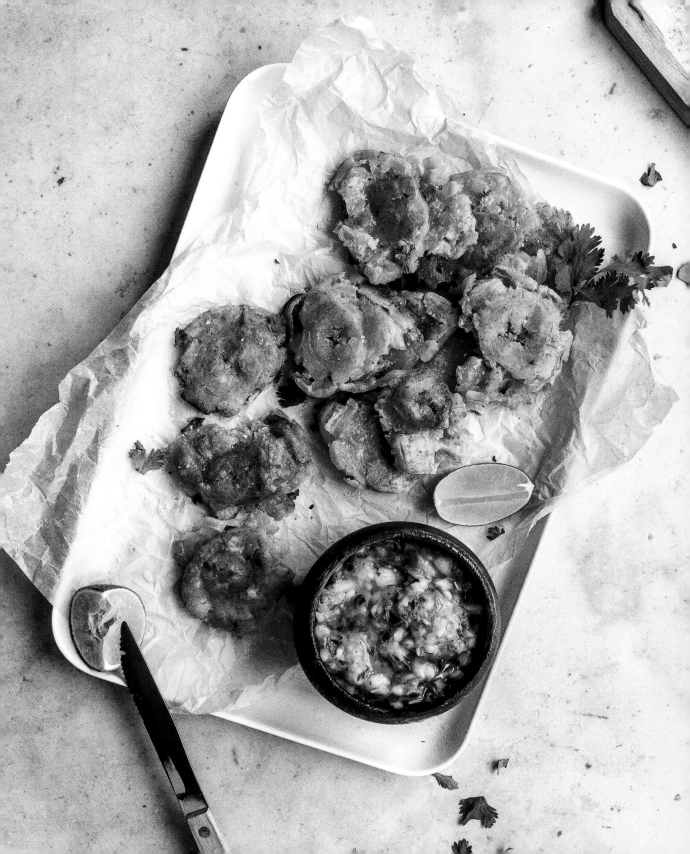

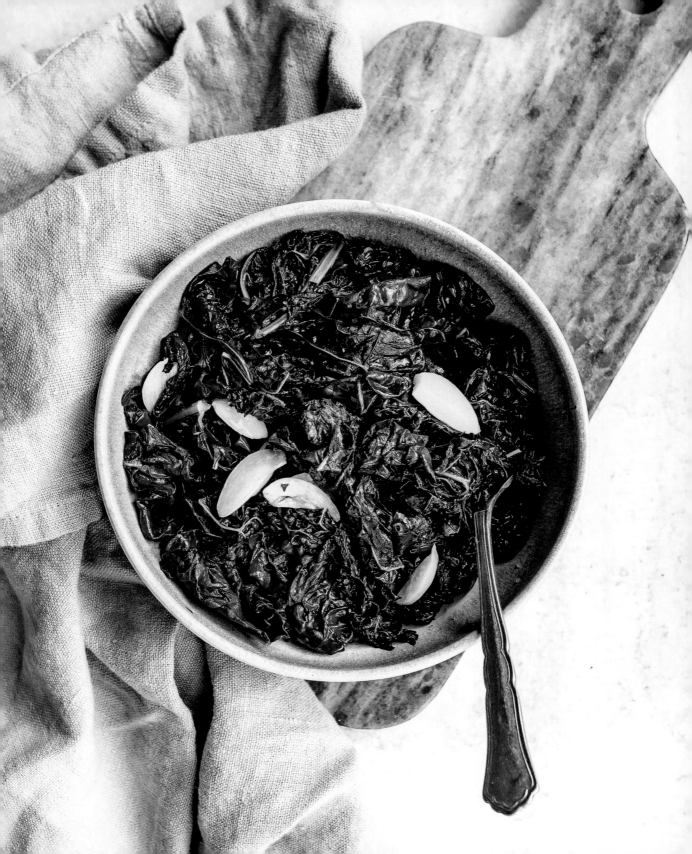

Bone Broth Garlic Kale

This gem of a recipe is simple and a permanent side staple in my house. It's one of my favorite ways to eat kale. After you try it, you'll have a hard time not making it constantly, too!

PREP TIME 5 minutes
COOK TIME 20 minutes
TOTAL TIME 25 minutes
YIELD 4 servings

3 tablespoons (45 ml) extra-virgin olive oil

3 cloves garlic, sliced into quarters

2 large bunches lacinato (dino) kale, de-stemmed

⅓ cup (30 ml) basic broth or bone broth, store-bought or homemade (page 182-183)

½ teaspoon sea salt

In a large skillet, heat the oil over medium-low heat. Add the garlic and cook for 1 to 2 minutes. Add the kale leaves and toss with tongs. Get the kale coated fully in the oil so it's nice and shiny. Raise the heat to medium as you toss for 1 to 2 minutes.

Add the broth and salt. Reduce the heat to low, cover, and cook for 15 to 20 minutes. It's done when the garlic is soft and all leaves are nice and tender.

Recipe Tip

You can use curly kale. I just find it much bulkier and more of a hassle to coat and sauté versus the dino kale.

Crispy Baked Sweet Potato Fries

Another delicious go-to side that's no-fuss. The easiest way to get crispy baked fries is to use a wire baking grate on top of your baking sheet if you've got one! It allows the air to circulate so there are no soggy sides. If you don't have one, no worries. Just flip the fries halfway through.

PREP TIME 10 minutes
COOK TIME 40 minutes
TOTAL TIME 50 minutes
YIELD 4 servings

2–3 medium-large sweet potatoes, cut into ¼-inch (6-mm)-thick fries

2 tablespoons (30 ml) extra-virgin olive oil

1 teaspoon sea salt, divided

Low-sugar ketchup, beet ketchup (for AIP), or a chimichurri (page 191) or salsa verde (page 192) for dipping (optional)

If you have the time, soak the cut sweet potatoes in a bowl of cold water for 30 minutes. This helps to remove the excess potato starch and make them even crispier.

Preheat the oven to 425°F (220°C, or gas mark 7) and arrange a rack in the middle. Line a large baking sheet (or 2 medium baking sheets) with parchment paper. If you have one, place a wire rack on top of the baking sheet.

Pat the sweet potato fries dry with paper towels. Toss them in the oil until well-coated.

Add the fries to the baking sheet(s) in a single layer and sprinkle ½ teaspoon of salt. Distribute them evenly so they can get crispy.

If using the wire rack, bake for 30 to 40 minutes straight through. The timing depends on your oven, so watch them after the 30-minute mark. If you're cooking directly on the baking sheet, flip the fries with a spatula halfway through.

Once the fries are golden brown and crisp, remove from the oven and season with ½ teaspoon of salt. Optionally serve with your favorite sauce or a low-sugar ketchup or beet ketchup for AIP!

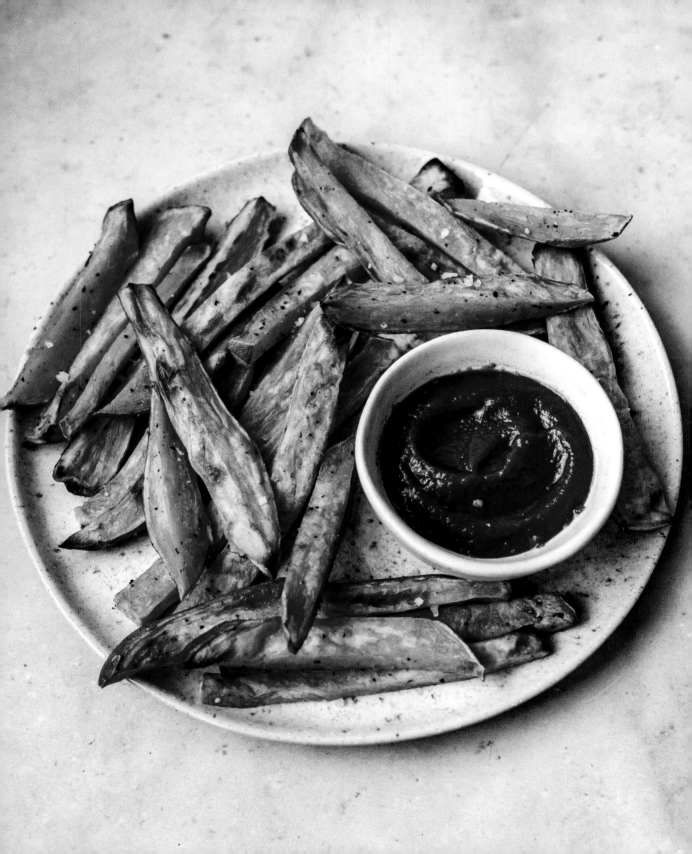

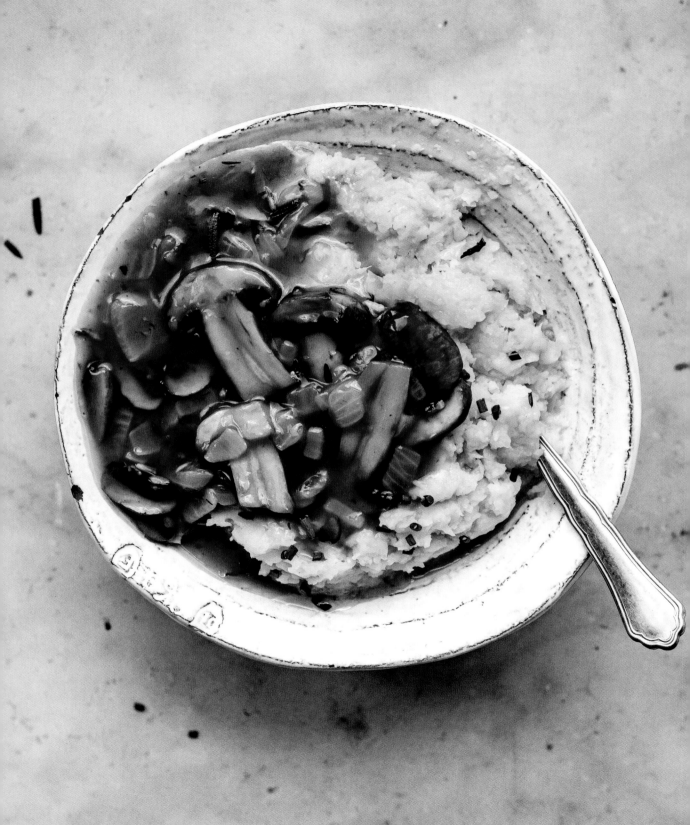

Creamy Mashed Cauliflower with Mushroom Gravy

This is one of my favorites, especially for the holidays, without the blood sugar spike and crash from traditional mashed potatoes. And you'll still get a similar creamy effect. The gravy made with earthy mushrooms, broth, and fresh herbs is tasty, and you might need to pour it on everything!

PREP TIME 10 minutes
COOK TIME 25 minutes
TOTAL TIME 35 minutes
YIELD 4 to 6 servings

MUSHROOM GRAVY
1 tablespoon (13 g) ghee or extra-virgin olive oil for AIP

1 small yellow onion or 2 shallots, chopped

10 ounces (280 g) cremini mushrooms, sliced thinly

2 tablespoons (18 g) arrowroot

2 cups (475 ml) basic broth or bone broth, store-bought or homemade (page 182 or 183)

3 sprigs of rosemary, de-stemmed and chopped

3 sprigs of thyme, de-stemmed and chopped

½ teaspoon sea salt

¼ teaspoon black pepper (omit for AIP)

MASHED CAULIFLOWER
2 cups (475 ml) water

2 heads of cauliflower, chopped into florets

2 tablespoons (30 ml) extra-virgin olive oil

¼ teaspoon sea salt

¼ teaspoon black pepper (omit for AIP)

To make the mushroom gravy: Heat a large skillet over medium heat. Add the ghee and melt, swirling to coat the bottom of the pan. Add the onion and stir with a wooden spoon for 2 to 3 minutes, until translucent. Add the mushrooms and continue to sauté for 5 minutes, until soft. Add a pinch of salt. Moisture should be releasing. Continue to stir until it evaporates.

Reduce the heat to low and sprinkle with the arrowroot. Continue to mix for 3 to 4 minutes, until a paste forms and turns golden. Slowly whisk in the broth, ensuring the starch is thickening it into gravy and any clumps are dissolved.

Add the herbs, salt, and pepper. Bring the gravy to a simmer for 7 to 8 minutes; it will continue to thicken. Continue to whisk until you are happy with the texture. It will continue to thicken even as it cools, so don't let it get too thick before removing from the heat!

To make the cauliflower: Bring water to boil, and place florets in a steam rack on top and cover. Steam for 7 to 8 minutes, until fork-tender but not falling apart. Alternatively, you may steam in the microwave for 3 to 4 minutes; do this in 2 to 3 batches in a bowl.

Add the florets to a food processor with the oil, salt, and pepper to taste. You may need to do this in batches. Alternatively, mash using a hand masher or an emulsion blender in a large mixing bowl or pot. Serve mashed cauliflower when smooth and pour mushroom gravy on top.

Irish Colcannon

A lower-carb option to the traditional Irish mashed potato dish using cauliflower and parsnips for an AIP Paleo side dish, this is perfect for your St. Paddy's table. Though, I encourage you to not wait for St. Paddy's Day to enjoy it!

PREP TIME 10 minutes
COOK TIME 25 minutes
TOTAL TIME 35 minutes
YIELD 4 servings

2 quarts (1.9 L) filtered water

½ teaspoon sea salt

2 pounds (907 g) parsnips, peeled, cored, and cut into 1-inch (2.5-cm) rounds

2 pounds (907 g) cauliflower, cut into florets

12 ounces (340 g) nitrate-free bacon, chopped

1 bunch lacinato "dino" kale, de-stemmed and chopped

1 bunch scallions, chopped

Olive oil or ghee (use olive oil for AIP)

Bring a large pot of salted water to a boil. Cook the parsnips for 8 minutes. Add the cauliflower florets and cook for 10 minutes, or until all veggies are fork-tender. Drain the vegetables and let them dry well.

Add the bacon to your pot over medium heat. Cook, stirring with a wooden spoon, for 8 minutes, until crispy. Add the kale and scallions and cook, stirring, for 2 to 3 minutes, until wilted. Set aside.

To a large serving bowl, add the parsnips and cauliflower and use a masher to mash them well. Alternatively, you could add them to a food processor and pulse until smooth.

Mix the bacon and kale in with your veggies in the serving bowl. Serve with a drizzle of olive oil.

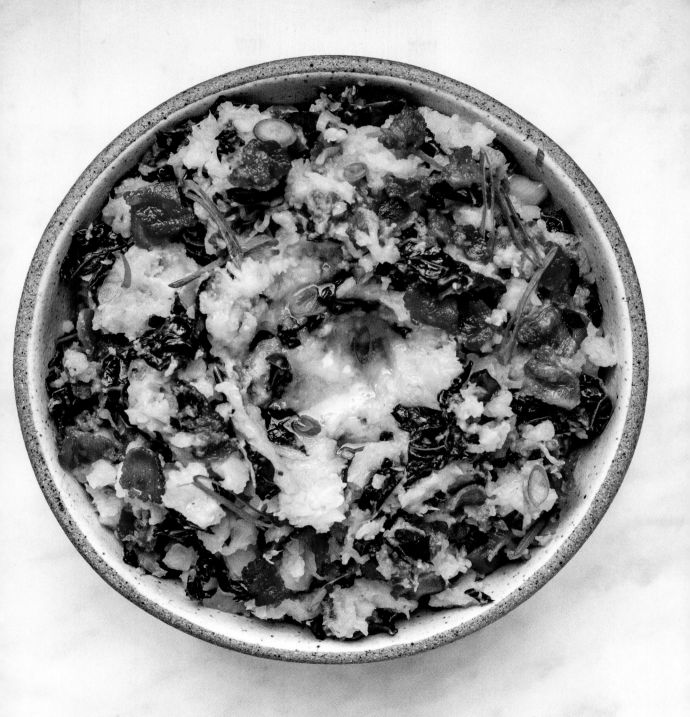

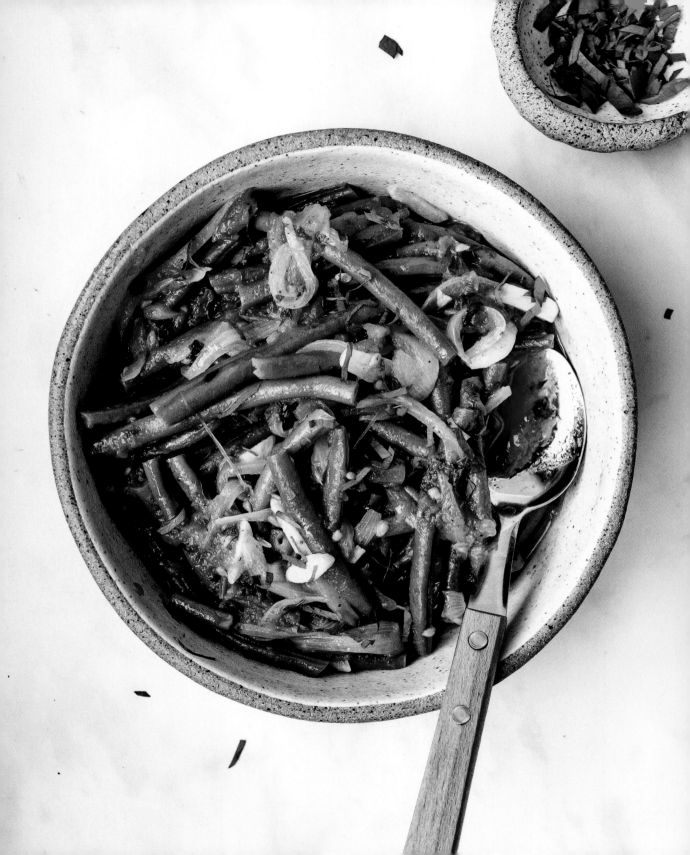

Fasolakia *(Haricots Verts in Tomato Sauce)*

Low-and-slow braising normally involves meat, but we're doing it to veggies. I can't stress how underrated this is! It takes a while to cook, but it's kind of a "set it and forget it" situation. This makes a great meal prep dish and gets tastier as it sits in the delicious broth. True story: This Greek family recipe from my husband's family got me loving green beans! If you're on AIP, bookmark this recipe for later when you can enjoy green beans and tomatoes.

PREP TIME 10 minutes
COOK TIME 50 minutes
TOTAL TIME 1 hour
YIELD 4 servings

¼ cup (59 ml) extra-virgin olive oil

1 yellow onion, sliced thinly

5 cloves garlic, sliced thinly

½ cup (30 g) chopped parsley (mostly leaves, some stems)

½ teaspoon sea salt

¼ teaspoon black pepper

1 pound (454 g) green beans (haricots verts), trimmed

2 large tomatoes, peeled and pureed in a food processor or finely chopped

3½ cups (825 ml) filtered water

To a large stockpot, add the oil over low-medium heat. Sauté the onion and garlic for about 5 minutes, until soft. Add the parsley and stir for 30 seconds. Season with salt and pepper.

Stir in the green beans and tomato until incorporated. Stir in the water. Cover the pot, reduce the heat to low, and let cook for 45 minutes or up to an hour, until the liquid has formed a brothy sauce and green beans are tender.

Recipe Tip

Skip this dish on the elimination phase of AIP due to the tomatoes and green beans.

Bone Broth Mangú with Salsa Verde

Mangú is a classic Dominican plantain dish that's easy, tasty, and filled with that good prebiotic starch. It has almost a mashed potato–type consistency with more oomph, and it's traditionally served with sautéed red onions. Here I'm being cheeky and using that delicious salsa verde (page 192) to top it off. Usually, the starchy water is mixed in to make the fluffy mash, but we're using bone broth for extra nutrient density!

PREP TIME 10 minutes
COOK TIME 20 minutes
TOTAL TIME 30 minutes
YIELD 4 to 6 servings

3 green unripe plantains

1 teaspoon sea salt, divided

2 bay leaves

¾ cup (175 ml) bone broth, store-bought or homemade (page 183)

1 tablespoon (15 ml) extra-virgin olive oil

1 teaspoon onion powder

1 teaspoon garlic powder

¼ teaspoon black pepper (omit for AIP)

1 batch of salsa verde (page 192)

Cut the ends off the plantains. Then cut them lengthwise and remove the green peel off by hand. Chop the plantains into thirds.

To a large pot, add the plantains, enough filtered water to cover, ½ teaspoon salt, and the bay leaves. Bring to a boil over high heat and cook for about 20 minutes, until fork-tender.

In a small saucepan, heat bone broth on a low simmer and then keep it covered and off the heat.

Remove the pot with the plantains from the heat, but don't drain it. Discard bay leaves. Using a slotted spoon, remove the plantains and add them to a large mixing bowl. Spoon in ½ cup (120 ml) of bone broth over the plantains. With a potato masher, mash the plantains. Season the mixture with onion powder, garlic powder, salt, and pepper.

The plantain mash will thicken as it sits, so keep it moving, continuing to mash and adding in the rest of the bone broth, pouring and mashing until you have the desired consistency.

When you're done adding the bone broth, you can use the hot starchy water if needed to loosen. It's up to you! Serve the mangú with a spoonful of salsa verde to taste. If you have leftovers, the mashed plantains will become more solid as they sit and cool. Simply reconstitute with a little water or broth when reheating and you'll be all set

Note: Plantains are high in prebiotic starch, and when that's new to your diet (aside from french fries), less is more. Common complaints of eating excess prebiotic veggies such as plantains, potatoes, or artichokes include gas and bloating. To reduce and eliminate that, start with small portions and work your way up over a few weeks until reaching a full portion that makes you feel good. Also, using bay leaves here (a carminative) helps to reduce and alleviate these symptoms, too! We do want to include prebiotic veggies in the diet in moderation to feed good bacteria in our guts.

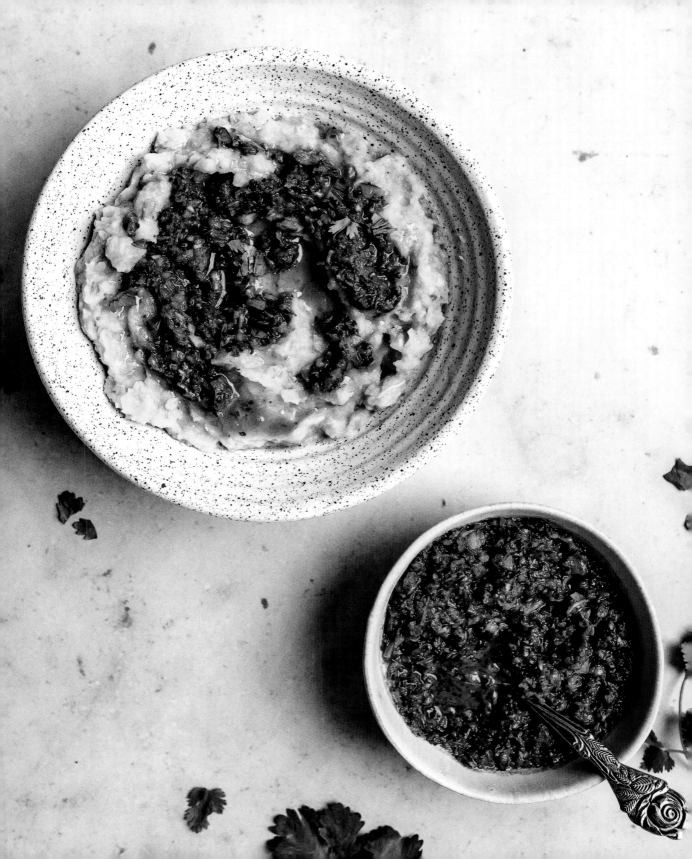

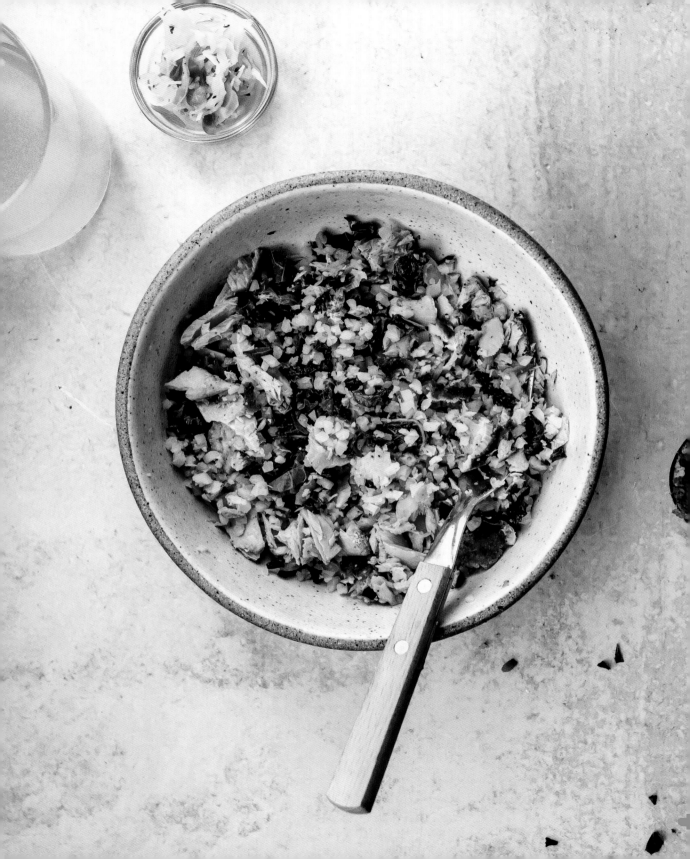

Veggie Confetti Rice

Plain cauliflower rice is quick and versatile, but I love to make rice from other vegetables (i.e., plantain rice, page 83). In this recipe, we're mixing cauliflower rice with sweet potato rice and some finely chopped kale, too. This is a great way to get three veggies all in one dish, and it's also the quickest way to cook these vegetables by far. The more variety of vegetables in your diet, the better for microbiome diversity—and more vitamins, minerals, and phytonutrients, too. Win-win!

PREP TIME 10 minutes
COOK TIME 10 minutes
TOTAL TIME 20 minutes
YIELD 4 servings

1 large sweet potato, peeled and chopped

1 tablespoon (15 ml) extra-virgin olive oil

1 bunch curly kale, de-stemmed and chopped

16 ounces (455 g) cauliflower rice

½ teaspoon sea salt

1 teaspoon garlic powder

½ teaspoon dried oregano

¼ teaspoon black pepper (omit for AIP)

Add the sweet potatoes to a food processor in a single layer. Do this in batches if necessary. Pulse until a "rice" forms. Set aside.

Heat the oil in a large skillet over medium heat. Add the kale and sauté for 1 to 2 minutes to wilt. Add the sweet potato and cauliflower rice. Add the seasonings and continue to cook, stirring, for 6 minutes, until well combined and everything is fork-tender.

Ginger Balsamic Beets and Greens

I hated beets, until I had them prepared along with their beautiful greens with balsamic vinegar. It's now something I could eat by the bowlful! Try it if you don't believe me. These are delicious served right away and hot, and they make tasty leftovers and match well with any salad!

PREP TIME 10 minutes

COOK TIME 1 hour and 10 minutes

TOTAL TIME 1 hour and 20 minutes

YIELD 4 servings

BEETS & GREENS

1 pound (454 g) beets with greens attached (3–4 medium)

1 teaspoon white vinegar

1 teaspoon sea salt, divided

2 teaspoons extra-virgin olive oil, divided

1 clove garlic, finely chopped

1 teaspoon minced ginger or ¼ teaspoon powder

¼ teaspoon black pepper (omit for AIP)

1 teaspoon balsamic vinegar

Chopped herbs, seeds, or nuts (optional; omit seeds/nuts for AIP)

BALSAMIC REDUCTION

¼ cup (60 ml) balsamic vinegar

1 tablespoon (6 g) minced ginger or 1 teaspoon powder

To make the beets: Chop the stems off, leaving a couple of inches attached. Add the whole beets to a large stockpot. Cover with cool filtered water. Add white vinegar and ½ teaspoon salt. Bring to a boil over medium-high heat. Once boiling, leave them at medium heat for 45 minutes to 1 hour, until fork-tender.

Prep the greens by snipping and discarding the stems; you can leave an inch or so on the ends of the leaves. Rinse the greens and let dry. Set aside.

Once beets are done, remove them from the water and place them on a cutting board. Add the greens to the hot water over low heat to blanch for 2 to 3 minutes, then set aside. You can discard the pink water now!

When the beets are cool enough to handle, get some kitchen gloves on and peel the outer layer off the beets and discard. Let the beets continue to cool.

To make the balsamic reduction: Add all the ingredients to a skillet over medium heat. Reduce, stirring occasionally with a spoon, for about 5 minutes. Watch it so it doesn't burn; don't be tempted to multitask.

Keep stirring until you see tiny bubbles form and you feel the vinegar get thicker. Once it's almost like a syrup, pour into a cup and set aside.

In that same skillet, add 1 teaspoon of oil and heat over low-medium. Add your greens and sauté for 2 to 3 minutes. Add the garlic, ½ teaspoon salt, ginger, and pepper. Cook and stir for 3 minutes, until the greens are dark. Plate the greens and grab all that leftover vinegar on the pan too!

Chop the beets into wedges and place them on top of the greens. Add the remaining oil and 1 teaspoon of vinegar, and lightly mix. Drizzle with balsamic reduction. Season with salt and garnish with herbs, seeds, or nuts.

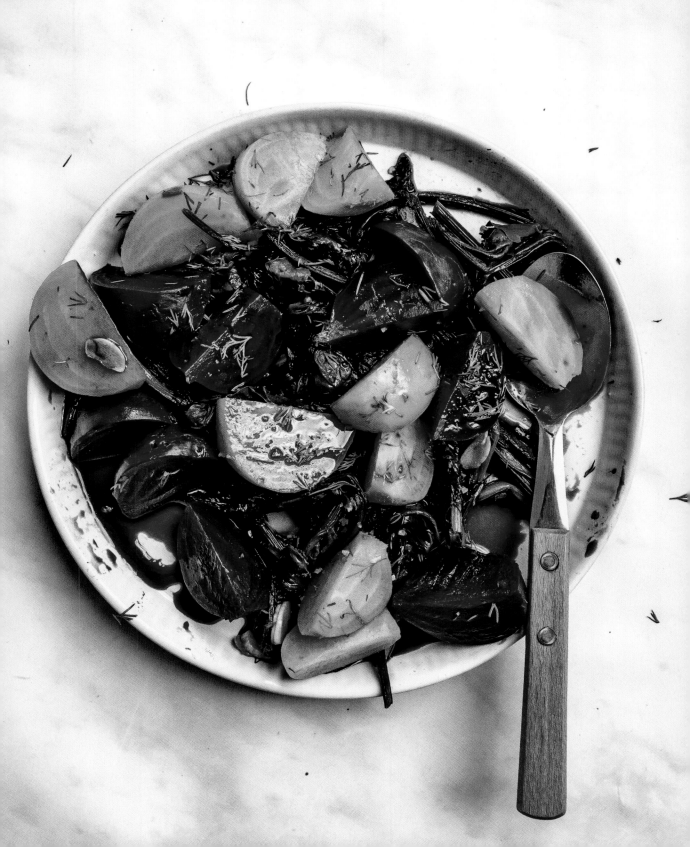

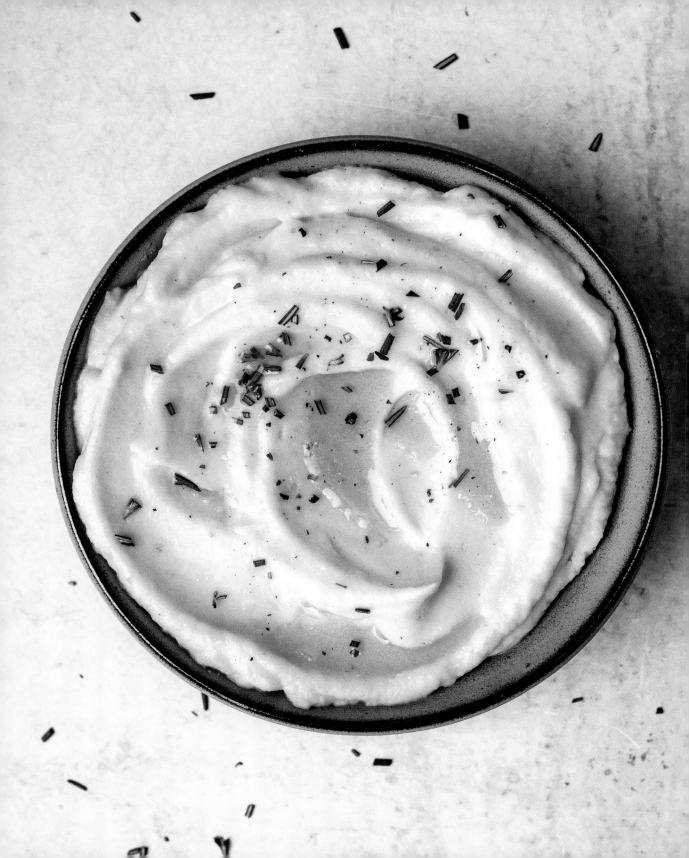

Rosemary Parsnip Puree

The more quick and easy sides, the better, am I right? I love the earthy, nutty taste of parsnips. This creamy preparation rounds out that extra bite parsnips have. Using this recipe as a base or side dish tastes delicious. It also has a very restaurant-esque presentation vibe going for it! You chef, you.

PREP TIME 10 minutes
COOK TIME 15 minutes
TOTAL TIME 25 minutes
YIELD 4 to 6 servings

4–5 cups (940 ml to 1.2 L) filtered water

1½ teaspoons sea salt, divided

1½ pounds (680 g) parsnips, peeled, cored, and cut in 1-inch (2.5-cm) rounds

½ cup (120 ml) full-fat unsweetened coconut milk, divided (additive-free for AIP)

3 tablespoons (39 g) ghee or extra-virgin olive oil (use olive oil for AIP)

1 tablespoon (2 g) chopped rosemary or 1 teaspoon dried, plus more for garnish

1 teaspoon sea salt

½ teaspoon black pepper (omit for AIP)

In a large stockpot, bring the water and ½ teaspoon salt to a boil. Cook the parsnips for 15 to 20 minutes, until fork-tender. Drain the parsnips in a colander in the sink for 2 or 3 minutes to fully drain and dry. Excess water in the puree will make it watery.

Using an emulsion (hand-held) blender: Rinse and dry off your pot. Add the drained parsnips back to the pot and pour in ¼ cup (60 ml) of coconut milk, ghee, rosemary, 1 teaspoon of salt, and pepper. Using the emulsion blender, hand-blend the mixture and taste. Add in coconut milk for a creamier consistency and season to taste.

Using a food processor: In batches, spoon out the drained parsnips and add them to the food processor in a single layer. Pulse until a puree forms. Once all parsnips have been pulsed, add to a large mixing bowl and mix in ¼ cup (60 ml) of coconut milk, ghee, rosemary, 1 teaspoon of salt, and pepper. Using a large spoon or potato masher, mix everything together. Add in the coconut milk for a creamier consistency to your liking and season more to taste.

Garnish with more rosemary (if using) and serve.

Gut Power Up

Top with some fermented veggies such as sauerkraut or Fermented Coleslaw (page 184) or, in place of coconut milk, you can always use coconut yogurt (or half of each) for more probiotics in your life!

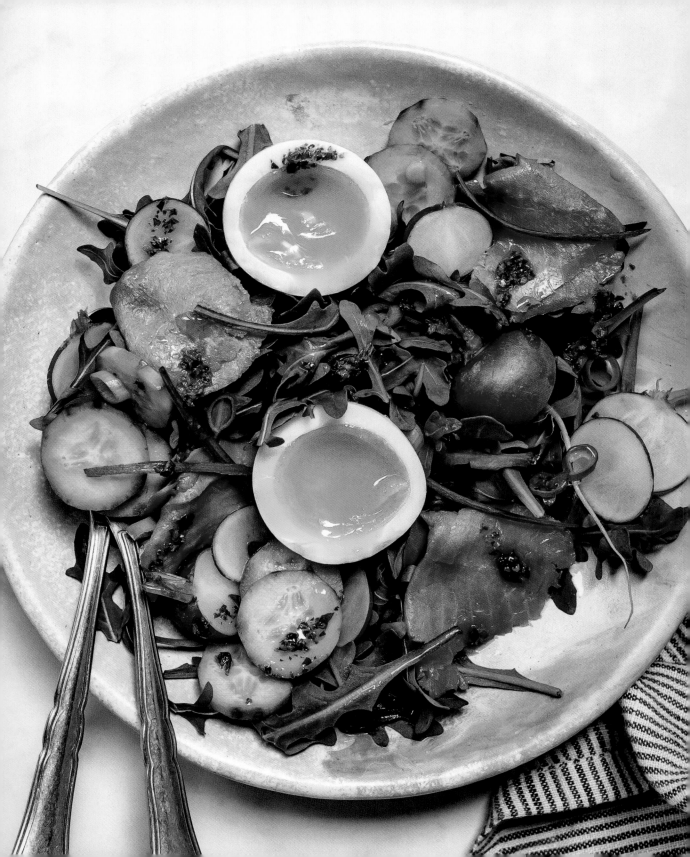

6

SALADS

In the warmer months especially, I just want a bowl of crunchy vegetables and easy proteins, all drizzled in some tasty dressing—even for breakfast, with some jammy eggs or wild smoked salmon (see page 148 for that recipe!). This is a collection of some of my favorite salads you can either prep or make on the fly, for one or for a crowd. I love making salads for potlucks because they can feed an army with little work and travel well! I'm also known to have a large bowl of massaged kale in the fridge all year round: It's easier to digest when massaged, lasts well in the fridge, and can be eaten as a salad or sautéed in just a few minutes.

Massaged Kale Caesar 140
Tuna Niçoise Salad 143
Tropical Shrimp Salad 144
Chicken Pad Thai with Green Papaya Noodles 147
Smoked Salmon Salad with Jammy Eggs 148

Massaged Kale Caesar

I used to eat a dairy-free kale Caesar salad in a café in the Lower East Side of Manhattan almost daily! It was a small hole-in-the-wall type of place called El Rey. Ever since, I've tried making my own variation at home. This is my spin on this beautiful, filling salad topped with shredded chicken (page 74), a boiled egg, and other fixings. It's a fabulous meal-prep salad because kale is so sturdy and gets even tastier as it sits.

PREP TIME 10 minutes
COOK TIME 10 minutes
TOTAL TIME 20 minutes
YIELD 4 servings

SALAD
3–4 cups (201–268 g) organic curly kale, de-stemmed and chopped into bite-size pieces

1 tablespoon (15 ml) extra-virgin olive oil

½ teaspoon sea salt

AVOCADO CAESAR DRESSING
1 small ripe avocado, pitted and peeled

2 cloves garlic, minced

3 anchovy fillets

1 tablespoon (15 g) Dijon mustard (omit for AIP)

1 tablespoon (15 ml) extra-virgin olive oil

Juice of 1 lemon

½ teaspoon sea salt

¼ teaspoon black pepper (omit for AIP)

1–2 tablespoons filtered water, as needed

TOPPINGS
4 soft-boiled eggs, peeled and sliced in half (omit for AIP)

2 cups (280 g) cooked and cooled shredded chicken (page 74)

1 small ripe avocado, sliced

¼ cup (60 g) Fermented Coleslaw (page 184) or sauerkraut

2–3 radishes, sliced

Chopped almonds, pepitas, crushed plantain, or sweet potato chips (omit nuts/seeds for AIP; optional)

To make the salad: Add the kale and oil to a large bowl. Massage the oil into the kale with your hands for 3 to 4 minutes, until the kale is soft and has reduced in size. Season with salt.

To make the dressing: Add all the ingredients to a blender or food processor. Blend until smooth. Adjust the seasonings and add water to loosen until you've reached a dressing consistency.

Lightly dress the kale and toss. Place the dressed salad in serving bowls and add eggs, chicken, avocado, coleslaw, radishes, and garnishes (if using).

Recipe Tip

Prepping components of this dish in advance makes for a quick and satisfying dish at lunch or dinner, and the massaged kale can also be prepared in advance, stored in the fridge in an airtight container for up to 6 days.

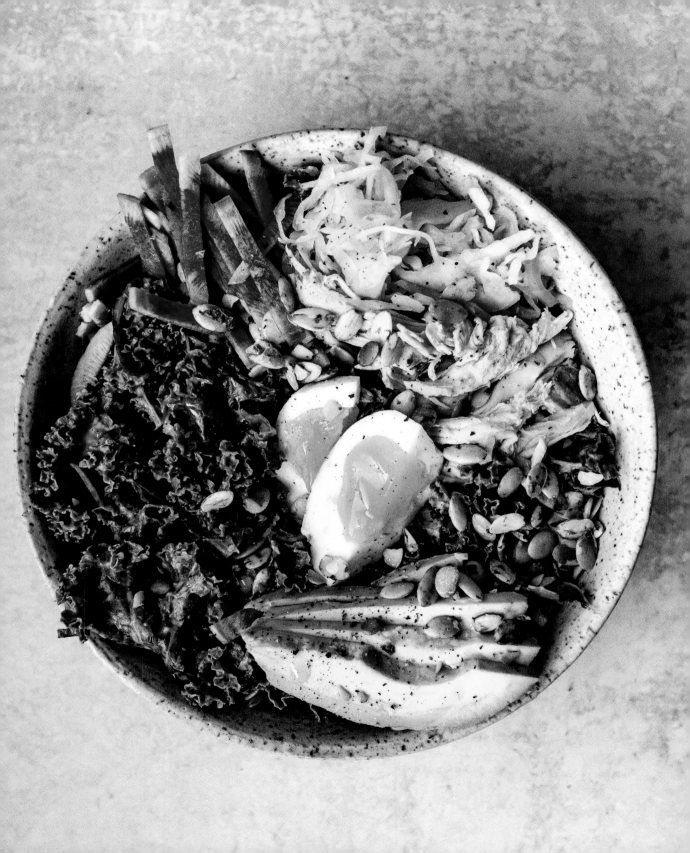

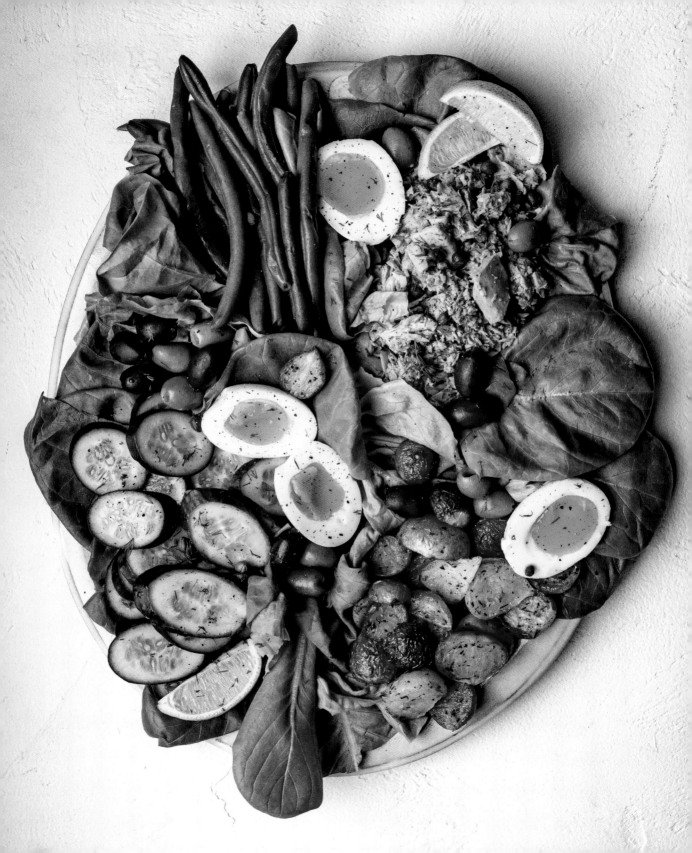

Tuna Niçoise Salad

I was lucky enough to visit Paris and enjoy an authentic tuna Niçoise salad with tasty extra-virgin olive oil, a pinch of herbes de Provence, and fresh vegetables. In place of the traditional baby potatoes, I'm subbing in roasted radishes. They are absolutely delicious and give a similar effect with a lot less of a blood sugar spike!

PREP TIME 10 minutes
COOK TIME 20 minutes
TOTAL TIME 30 minutes
YIELD 4 servings

SALAD

1 pound (454 g) radishes, ends trimmed and halved

1 tablespoon (15 ml) extra-virgin olive oil

½ teaspoon sea salt

¼ teaspoon garlic powder

4 soft-boiled eggs, peeled and sliced in half (omit for AIP)

2 (4.5-ounce, or 128-g) cans tuna in water, drained (tongol or skipjack recommended for lower mercury levels)

1 cup (100 g) green beans (sub spinach or asparagus for AIP)

½ English cucumber or 2 mini cucumbers, chopped

4 cups (220 g) butter lettuce, torn

⅓ cup (33 g) pitted Kalamata olives

2 teaspoons capers

¼ teaspoon sea salt

LEMON DRESSING

Juice of 2 lemons

Zest from 1 lemon

⅓ cup (79 ml) extra-virgin olive oil

1 teaspoon Dijon mustard (sub 1 teaspoon apple cider vinegar for AIP)

1 teaspoon raw honey

½ teaspoon sea salt

½ teaspoon dried herbes de Provence (optional)

To make the salad: Preheat the oven to 425°F (220°C, or gas mark 7) and line a baking sheet with parchment paper. Add the radishes and toss with oil, salt, and garlic powder. Spread out in a single layer and roast for 20 to 25 minutes, until golden and crisp on the outside and fork-tender on the inside. Remove from the oven and set aside to come to room temperature.

To make the dressing: Combine the ingredients in a food processor and pulse until combined.

Place the lettuce in a bowl and toss with 2 to 3 tablespoons of dressing. Arrange the remaining ingredients on top of the lettuce and drizzle more dressing on top. Finish with a pinch of salt.

Tropical Shrimp Salad

This is a salad that will make you think you're on vacation: tropical flavors from mango salsa (page 193), avocado crema dressing, and grilled shrimp. And it's oh so easy to make! Swap the shrimp for shredded chicken (page 74) or serve with pork chops, which pair so well with mango. Or even crush plantain chips on top—it's a delicious addition.

PREP TIME 10 minutes
COOK TIME 10 minutes
TOTAL TIME 20 minutes
YIELD 4 servings

SHRIMP

2 pounds (907 g) frozen or fresh shrimp, peeled and deveined

2 tablespoons (30 ml) extra-virgin olive oil, divided

½ teaspoon sea salt

¼ teaspoon black pepper (omit for AIP)

½ teaspoon paprika (omit for AIP)

½ teaspoon dried coriander (omit for AIP)

AVOCADO CREMA DRESSING

1 small avocado, pitted and peeled

2 tablespoons (20 g) chopped red onion

Juice of ½ lime

3 tablespoons (45 ml) extra-virgin olive oil, plus more as needed

¼ cup (4 g) chopped cilantro

½ teaspoon sea salt

SALAD

2 medium heads of butter or red leaf lettuce (or similar), washed and torn

½ batch mango salsa (page 193)

½ ripe mango, diced (from the mango salsa recipe)

2 mini cucumbers or ½ English cucumber, sliced

3–4 lime wedges for garnish (optional)

To make the shrimp: Toss thawed shrimp with 1 tablespoon (15 ml) of oil, salt, pepper, paprika, and coriander in a mixing bowl. Heat a large skillet or cast iron over medium heat and add 1 tablespoon (15 ml) of oil. Once shimmering, add the shrimp in a single layer with marinade. Cook for 1 to 2 minutes on each side, until pink and cooked through. Transfer the shrimp to a plate, and set aside.

To make the dressing: Combine all the ingredients in a food processor or blender. Pulse until well combined and smooth. Optionally loosen with more oil and season to taste. Pour the dressing into a small bowl.

To make the salad: To a large salad bowl, add the lettuce and lightly dress with 1 to 2 tablespoons of the dressing. Mix well. Arrange the shrimp on top of the lettuce and drizzle with the mango salsa. Top with mango pieces and cucumbers. Serve the remaining dressing alongside the salad, with lime wedges.

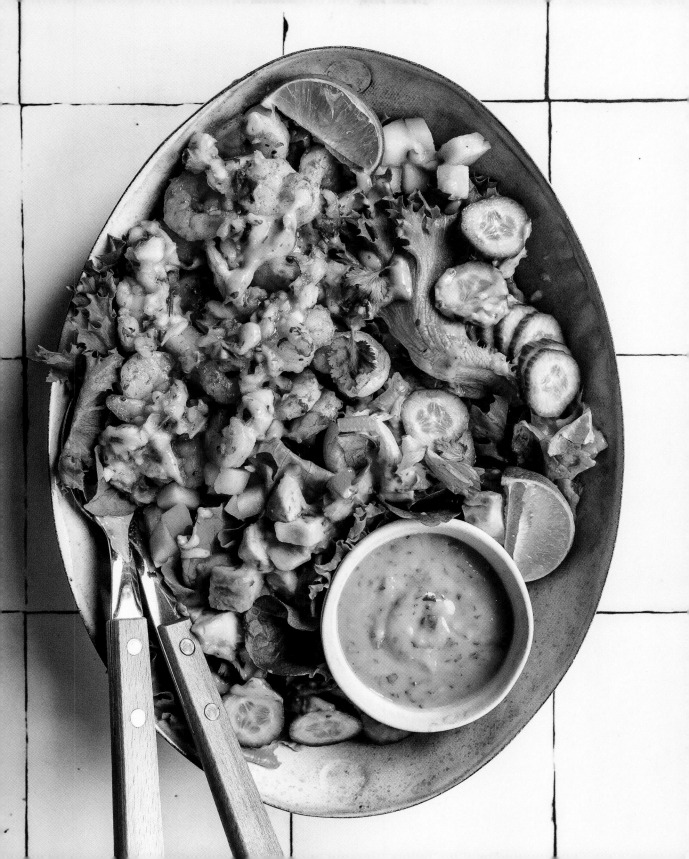

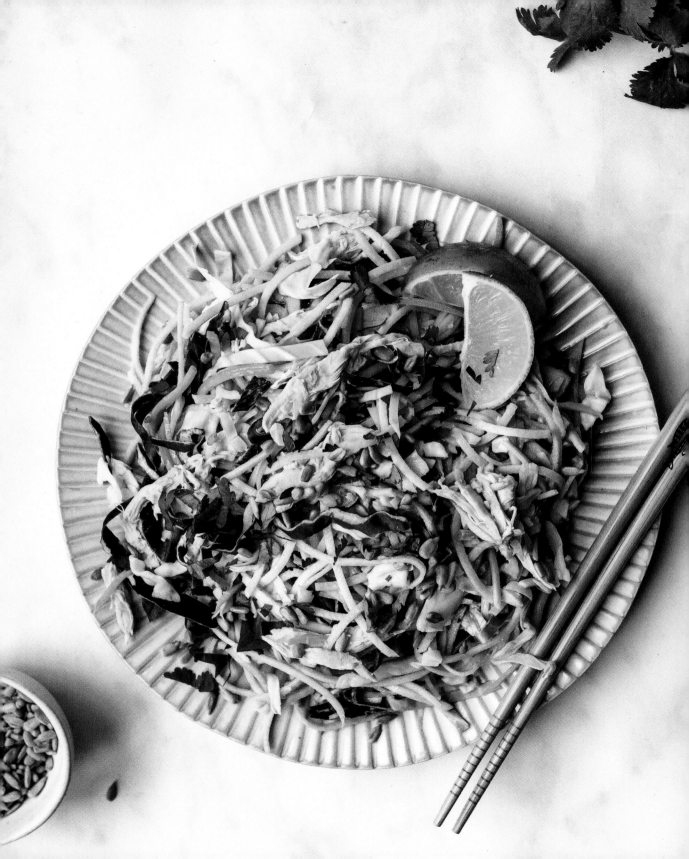

Chicken Pad Thai with Green Papaya Noodles

This bold salad has put my old Thai takeout habit to shame. The sauce uses sunflower seed butter and coconut aminos instead of traditional peanut butter and soy sauce, and the green papaya noodles are wonderful for gut health, with natural enzymes to aid in digestion! If you can't find papaya, zucchini noodles (zoodles) are a great substitute. For easier digestion, lightly sauté the noodles, cabbage, and carrots in 2 to 3 teaspoons (10 to 15 ml) of olive oil.

PREP TIME 10 minutes
COOK TIME 10 minutes
TOTAL TIME 20 minutes
YIELD 4 servings

SAUCE (see below for an AIP-friendly version)

⅓ cup (86 g) plain, unsweetened sunflower seed butter

¼ cup (60 ml) fresh lime juice

2 tablespoons (12 g) minced ginger or ginger juice

2 cloves garlic, minced

2 tablespoons (28 ml) coconut aminos

1 tablespoon (15 ml) toasted sesame oil

¼ teaspoon fish sauce

¼ teaspoon sea salt

3–4 tablespoons (45–60 ml) filtered water

AIP-FRIENDLY SAUCE

⅓ cup (79 ml) extra-virgin olive oil

¼ cup (60 ml) fresh lime juice

2 teaspoons raw honey

2 tablespoons (12 g) minced ginger

2 cloves garlic, minced

3 tablespoons (45 ml) coconut aminos

¼ teaspoon fish sauce

½ teaspoon sea salt

PAD THAI

⅓ cup (48 g) toasted sunflower seeds (optional; omit for AIP)

1 large green papaya, peeled, seeded, and spiralized

1 cup (110 g) shredded carrots

1 cup (70 g) thinly sliced cabbage

3–4 scallions, chopped

¼ cup (4 g) chopped cilantro, plus more for garnish

2 red bell peppers, sliced thinly (omit for AIP)

4 cups (560 g) shredded chicken breast (page 74)

1 lime, cut into 4 wedges

To make either sauce: Combine all the ingredients in a food processor. Pulse until smooth and set aside.

To make the pad Thai: If using, toast the sunflower seeds over a hot nonstick pan for 1 to 2 minutes while tossing frequently. Pay close attention so they don't burn! Set aside.

To assemble the salad: Toss all the veggies with the sauce in a large mixing bowl. Add the chicken and toss. Serve with toasted sunflower seeds, lime wedges, and more cilantro.

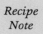

Recipe Note

Papaya is well known for its high content of vitamins C and A, carotenoids, and fiber, with a key enzyme called papain, which aids in the digestion of meat. Studies have shown it may reduce inflammatory markers. Green (unripe) papayas have less sugar and a higher concentration of the protein-digesting enzyme, papain, than the ripe ones.

Smoked Salmon Salad with Jammy Eggs

I love a good breakfast salad, and this one is bursting with flavor. This and a hot cup of bone broth or matcha, and I'm ready to go! Prep the dressing and eggs ahead of time for an easy weekday breakfast. I love doubling or tripling the delicious pesto to freeze.

PREP TIME 5 minutes
COOK TIME 10 minutes
TOTAL TIME 15 minutes
YIELD 4 servings

PESTO DRESSING
¼ cup extra-virgin olive oil

2 cups fresh basil

1 tablespoon nutritional yeast

1 teaspoon sea salt

1 garlic clove, chopped or minced

½ lemon, juiced

SALAD
4–6 cups (220–330 g) arugula or mixed greens

4 radishes, sliced thinly

3 mini cucumbers, sliced thinly

2 scallions, sliced thinly

8 ounces (225 g) wild smoked salmon (additive-free)

4 soft-boiled, pasture-raised eggs, sliced in half (sub more salmon, chicken, bacon, or prosciutto for AIP)

To make the pesto dressing: Combine all the ingredients in a food processor. Pulse until smooth. Add more oil if needed to reach the desired consistency.

To assemble the salad: In a large bowl, toss all veggies and greens with dressing. Add smoked salmon and eggs. Store any extra dressing in the fridge in an airtight container for up to 5 days or freeze in ice cube trays to always have some handy!

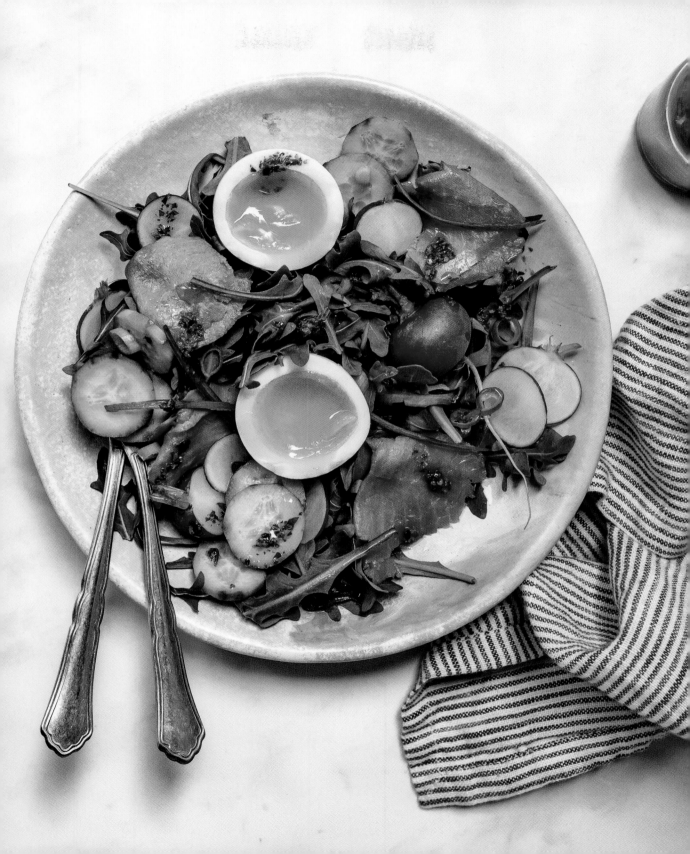

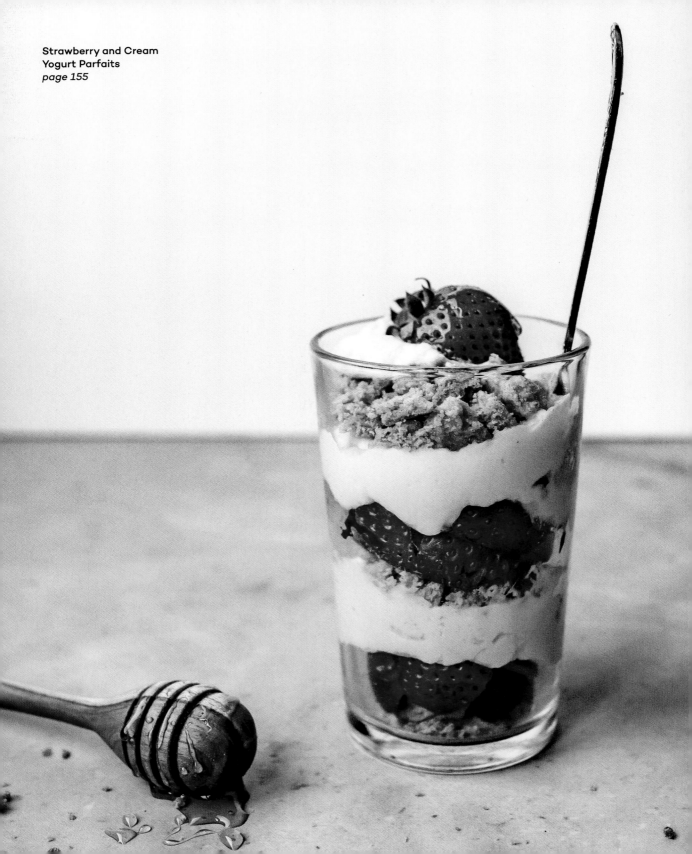

**Strawberry and Cream
Yogurt Parfaits**
page 155

7

DESSERTS

Eating Paleo transformed me from a Pop Tart addict to a self-proclaimed dark chocolate connoisseur. Fresh fruit, dark chocolate, some coconut, or nuts and I'm a happy gal. And as it turns out, you can get creative with those ingredients! These recipes are made from whole-food ingredients, most are AIP-friendly (or nut-free), and they will give you a great mix to satisfy any sweet tooth without the junk. I err on the low- to no-sweetener side, so adjust it to your taste. My philosophy on dessert is to eat it mindfully or not at all. It's meant to be a treat and you deserve to enjoy it!

Peach Cobbler 152
Sautéed Cinnamon Apples with Yogurt 154
Strawberry and Cream Yogurt Parfaits 155
Pineapple, Lime, and Mint Sorbet 156
No-Churn Blueberry Cardamom Nice Cream 157
Coconut Custard Pie 158
Tahini Caramel Bars 160
Cranberry Orange Flourless Muffins 163

Peach Cobbler

Baked fruit is one of my favorite desserts ever. Get creative with seasonal fruits such as apples, pears, and cranberries in the autumn and winter, and stone fruit or berries in the spring and summer. It's so easy to make with minimal fuss or mess, and it's a real crowd-pleaser. Use the Instant Pot Coconut Yogurt (page 187) to top for a little probiotic addition to your baked fruit or check out my blog for an AIP ice cream recipe!

PREP TIME 10 minutes
COOK TIME 30 minutes
TOTAL TIME 40 minutes
YIELD 4 servings

FILLING

4–5 medium semiripe or ripe peaches, pitted and sliced

1 tablespoon (9 g) arrowroot

Juice of ½ lemon

1 tablespoon (20 g) raw honey or maple syrup

½ teaspoon vanilla extract (alcohol-free for AIP)

¼ teaspoon ground cinnamon

¼ teaspoon ground cardamom (omit for AIP)

⅛ teaspoon sea salt

TOPPING

3 tablespoons (45 ml) avocado or coconut oil

½ cup (48 g) tigernut flour (for AIP) or almond flour, sifted

1 tablespoon (9 g) arrowroot

¼ teaspoon vanilla extract (alcohol-free for AIP)

1 tablespoon (20 g) raw honey or maple syrup

¼ teaspoon ground cinnamon

¼ teaspoon ground cardamom (omit for AIP)

¼ teaspoon sea salt

FOR SERVING

Store-bought or homemade Paleo vanilla ice cream, coconut yogurt (page 187), or whipped coconut cream (optional; use AIP-friendly)

To make the filling: Preheat the oven to 350°F (175°C, or gas mark 4).

Add the peaches to a baking dish or pie dish. I used a 6 x 4-inch (15 x 10-cm) dish. Add the arrowroot, lemon juice, honey, vanilla, spices, and salt. Stir to combine. Pat the filling down into a single even layer.

To make the topping: Add all the ingredients to a medium mixing bowl. Hand-mix using a spoon or fork until well combined. Smooth out into a single layer with a tablespoon. Use the tablespoon to scoop out the batter and form biscuit-like patties with your hands, ¼ inch (6 mm) thick. You want to cover your filling in a single layer, but leave enough room between them so they cook evenly.

Bake for 25 to 30 minutes, until golden brown and the filling is bubbling. Let sit for 5 to 10 minutes before serving. Top with Paleo ice cream, yogurt, or coconut whipped cream (if using).

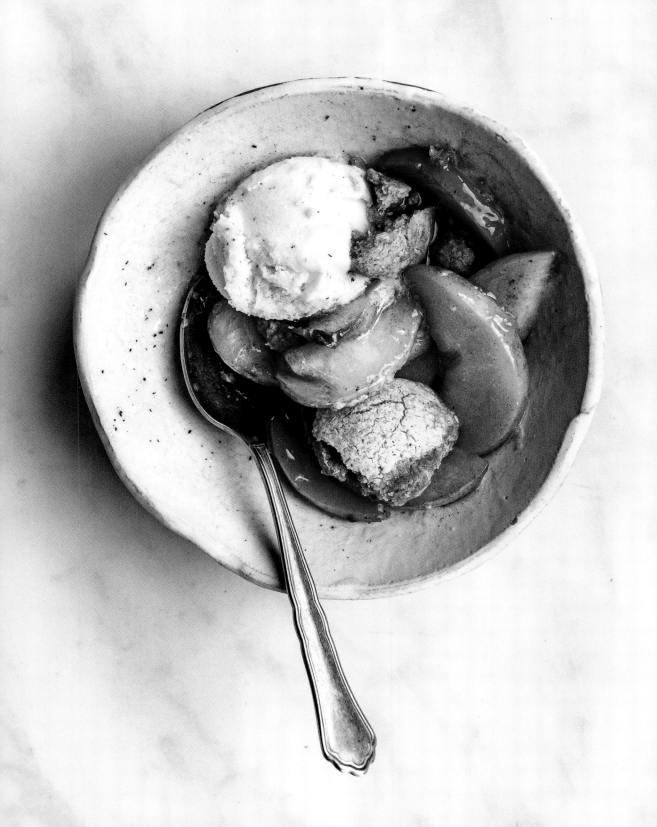

Sautéed Cinnamon Apples with Yogurt

Dessert is dessert, right? Nope! This combination of fruit, fat, and spices highlights how good for you a dessert can be! Similar to the Peach Cobbler (page 152), this is a dish that's easy to make and you can feel so good about enjoying solo or with loved ones, tea in hand, because it's nutritious and delicious. *Bon appétit!*

PREP TIME: 5 minutes
COOK TIME: 10 minutes
TOTAL TIME: 15 minutes
YIELD: 4 servings

4–6 large honey crisp apples

1 tablespoon (14 g) coconut oil for AIP or ghee

2 teaspoons maple syrup or raw honey, plus more to taste

1 tablespoon (15 ml) water

¼ teaspoon ground nutmeg, plus more to taste (omit for AIP)

1 teaspoon ground cinnamon, plus more to taste

¼ teaspoon ground cardamom, plus more to taste (omit for AIP)

¼ teaspoon sea salt

¼–½ cup (60–120 g) coconut yogurt (homemade, page 187, or additive-free for store-bought)

Peel the apples if you prefer. Core them and slice thinly, about ½ inch (1 cm) thick. Melt the coconut oil in a large skillet or cast-iron skillet over medium-low heat. Add the apple slices and maple syrup. Stir with a wooden spoon, then add the water and seasonings.

Continue to cook apples, stirring occasionally, until they're nice and soft after 7 to 8 minutes. Taste and adjust seasonings and or sweetener.

Let sit for at least 2 to 3 minutes off the heat, then serve with a dollop of coconut yogurt and a sprinkle of cinnamon. This will store well in an airtight container for 4 to 5 days in the fridge.

Strawberry and Cream Yogurt Parfaits

If you love strawberries and cream or strawberry shortcake, this combines both into a pretty and simple dessert with a healthy dose of probiotics. These make a great party dessert!

PREP TIME 10 minutes
COOK TIME 15 minutes
TOTAL TIME 25 minutes
YIELD 4 to 6 servings

COOKIE CRUMBLE

½ cup (56 g) cassava or coconut flour, sifted

¼ cup (20 g) unsweetened shredded coconut

¼ cup (59 ml) avocado or coconut oil

¼ teaspoon vanilla extract (alcohol-free for AIP)

1 tablespoon (20 g) raw honey or maple syrup

¼ teaspoon ground cinnamon

⅛ teaspoon sea salt

PARFAIT

1½ cups (249 g) strawberries, hulled and sliced ¼ inch (6 mm) thick

Juice of ½ lemon

2 tablespoons (40 g) raw honey or maple syrup

¼ teaspoon sea salt

24–36 ounces (680 g–1 kg) coconut yogurt (homemade, page xx or additive free for store-bought), 6 ounces (170 g) per person

Preheat the oven to 350°F (175°C, or gas mark 4) and line a baking sheet with parchment paper.

To make the crumble: Add all the ingredients to the food processor and pulse until a crumble forms. Spread it out on the baking sheet in a single layer using a spatula. Bake for 10 to 15 minutes, until golden brown. Remove and let sit and come to room temperature. When it's at room temperature, break it up into "crumbles."

To make the parfait: Mix the strawberries with lemon juice, honey, and salt. Using short drinking glasses, glass ramekins, or small jars, layer the parfait by adding a spoonful of cookie crumbles, followed by a spoonful of strawberries, followed by yogurt. Repeat the layers in order again and finish with a sprinkle of cookie crumbles.

These will store well if kept in airtight containers for up to 3 days if you'd like to prepare them in advance, or simply prepare the cookie crumbles and store those in the fridge to assemble it the day of.

Pineapple, Lime, and Mint Sorbet

Easy and refreshing, this dessert will cool you down—and cool your digestion, too! If you use fresh pineapple for this recipe, cut it into 1-inch (2.5-cm) chunks and freeze it for at least 4 hours. The magic of blending frozen fruit makes for a smooth sorbet with minimal ingredients. The sweetener takes some of the tart zing off, but you can always go without because of the pineapple's natural sugars! Pineapple is rich in vitamin C, manganese, and an enzyme called bromelain, a group of digestive enzymes that breaks down proteins. Pineapples are also loaded with healthy antioxidants that may aid in fighting chronic inflammation.

PREP TIME: 10 minutes
COOK TIME: 0 minutes
TOTAL TIME: 10 minutes
YIELD: 4 servings

2½ cups (413 g) frozen pineapple chunks

Juice and zest of 1 lime

1 teaspoon raw honey or maple syrup (optional)

2 tablespoons (12 g) chopped mint leaves

Add frozen pineapple to a food processor. Pulse until crumbles form. If you have a smaller food processor, you may need to do this in batches. Add the lime juice, lime zest, and honey (if using). Continue pulsing until everything is combined and the texture changes to a sorbet. If it's being difficult, add some filtered water by the tablespoon and pulse to help loosen. Garnish with mint leaves. You can freeze this in an airtight container for up to 1 week.

No-Churn Blueberry Cardamom Nice Cream

I eat this dessert regularly because it's super easy and satisfying, with no fuss or special equipment! You can adapt this with different flavors and types of frozen fruit using it as a template. You can also make it in batches to freeze in advance, but I mostly do it on the fly. Add probiotics by including a dollop of Instant Pot Coconut Yogurt (page 187) on top or in the mix!

PREP TIME 10 minutes
COOK TIME 0 minutes
TOTAL TIME 10 minutes
YIELD 2 servings

½ cup (78 g) frozen blueberries

½ cup (78 g) frozen cherries

1 heaping tablespoon (16 g) almond butter, cashew butter, or coconut cream

1 teaspoon raw honey or maple syrup (optional)

¼ teaspoon ground cardamom (sub ground cinnamon for AIP)

3–4 tablespoons (45–60 ml) nondairy milk, as needed (additive-free coconut milk for AIP)

Add all the ingredients, except the nondairy milk, to a food processor. Pulse until crumbles form.

Add 2 tablespoons (28 ml) of nondairy milk and continue to pulse until a smooth consistency forms. You can keep adding nondairy milk by the spoonful to loosen it up as needed. It will be thicker the less milk you use; you can also take 30-second breaks between pulsing to allow the frozen fruit to melt a bit.

You can make it in batches and store for up to 1 week in an airtight container in the freezer.

Make It AIP

Use coconut cream or coconut butter (manna) in place of nut butter. Use an AIP-friendly nondairy milk such as additive-free coconut or tigernut, and sub ground cinnamon for cardamom.

Coconut Custard Pie

My *abuelo* loved having this pie every Thanksgiving. We'd scour the grocery store Entenmann's display case to find the perfect one. It was always a special treat because nuts and coconuts were a no-go in my house (Mom's allergic). So, he and I would sneak off just far away enough from the dining room to enjoy it together. This Paleo/AIP version transports me right back to a simpler time with my loved and lost ones!

PREP TIME 20 minutes
COOK TIME 30 minutes
TOTAL TIME 2 hours to overnight
YIELD 8 to 10 servings

PIE CRUST

½ cup (102 g) tallow or leaf lard

1 teaspoon coconut oil or olive oil for greasing

1 cup (140 g) cassava flour

¼ teaspoon fine sea salt

2 tablespoons (28 ml) full-fat additive-free coconut milk, chilled but not solid

¼–½ cup (60–120 ml) filtered ice water, as needed

FILLING

1½ cups (120 g) unsweetened shredded coconut

1 medium white sweet potato, peeled and chopped into 1-inch pieces (about ¾–1 cup)

2 cups (475 ml) filtered water

1 can (13.5 ounce, or 383 g) full-fat coconut milk

¾ tablespoon (7 g) grass-fed gelatin powder

3 tablespoons (45 ml) maple syrup or raw honey

Coconut yogurt (page 187) or additive-free whipped coconut cream (optional)

If using leaf lard, measure ½ cup and drop it in tablespoons on a plate, then store it in the refrigerator to get cold until ready for use in the pie crust for at least 15 minutes. If using tallow, you don't need to refrigerate it, as it's hard enough.

Preheat the oven to 375°F (190°C, or gas mark 5). Line a baking sheet with parchment paper. Spread the shredded coconut in a single layer on the sheet and toast for 3 to 5 minutes, stirring once, until the coconut is golden and fragrant. Keep a close watch and remove promptly, transferring it to a plate when done. Set aside.

To make the crust: Lightly grease a 9-inch (23-cm) pie dish with coconut oil. To a food processor, combine flour, salt, and 1 to 2 spoonfuls of the tallow. Pulse until incorporated. Keep adding in the spoonfuls of tallow one at a time and pulsing until crumbly. Pour the mixture into a bowl. Add the chilled coconut milk; it shouldn't be solid or a "cream" (stir, if needed). Mix by hand and add ice water 1 tablespoon (15 ml) at a time as you form the dough into a ball. Only use as much water as needed to form a ball.

To your workspace, add a sheet of parchment paper and set aside a second piece for rolling. Sprinkle 1 to 2 teaspoons of cassava flour on the parchment paper. Add the dough ball on top with the parchment paper. Roll out the dough in a circular motion using a rolling pin, until it's about ⅛ inch (3 mm) thick. Transfer to your pie dish and lightly press the dough evenly against the dish, doing any "surgery" needed to make it look presentable! With a fork, lightly poke the bottom of the dough a few times evenly around. Bake for 25 to 30 minutes, until flaky and crisp. Set aside to cool.

To make the filling: Boil the peeled and diced white sweet potato in enough water to cover, until fork-tender. Drain and let cool for 10 minutes. Pour the coconut milk into a medium bowl and add the gelatin, whisking until well-combined. Let sit or "bloom" for 15 minutes.

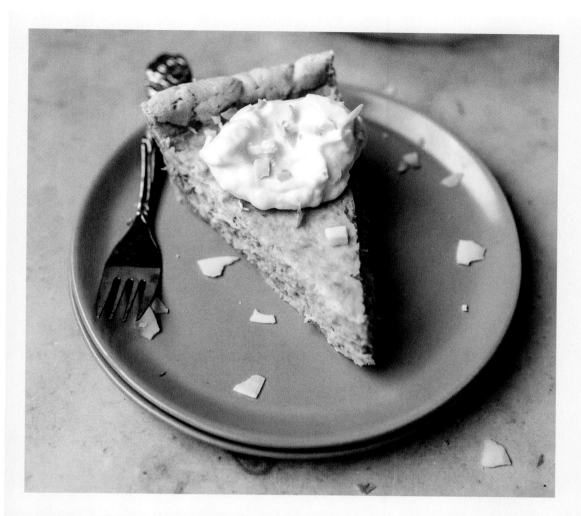

With a fork, mash the sweet potato and add to a high-speed blender. Add in the coconut milk—gelatin mixture, and syrup. Blend for 20 seconds or so until smooth. Pour the mixture back into a mixing bowl and using a spatula, fold in the toasted coconut until well combined.

Pour the custard mixture into the room temperature pie crust evenly and place in the refrigerator to set for at least 2 hours or overnight. Once the pie is set and the filling has thickened, remove from the refrigerator and let it come to room temperature (about 1 hour). Serve with a dollop of coconut yogurt or whipped coconut cream (if using). Store in an airtight container in the refrigerator for up to 1 week.

Tahini Caramel Bars

These homemade Twix bars made with tahini are a reader favorite for good reason. The shortbread cookie crust piled high with a date-based caramel and tahini is a killer combo, smothered in melted chocolate to top it all off. You can use another nut or seed butter; the flavor will be different, but still delicious and Twix-like. I store them in the freezer to pick at, not that they last very long!

PREP TIME 30 minutes
COOK TIME 12 minutes
TOTAL TIME 42 minutes
YIELD 8 servings

SHORTBREAD COOKIE CRUST

½ cup (48 g) tigernut flour

3 tablespoons (45 ml) avocado or melted coconut oil

2 tablespoons (30 ml) maple syrup

TAHINI CARAMEL FILLING

5 soaked dates

2 cups (475 ml) boiling water

¼ cup (60 g) tahini or tigernut butter for an AIP substitute

½ teaspoon vanilla extract (alcohol-free for AIP)

Pinch sea salt

TOPPING

⅓ cup (58 g) chopped dark chocolate (Paleo-friendly; 85% cacao and above recommended) (see AIP notes)

1 tablespoon (15 ml) coconut oil

Flaky sea salt

Soak the dates in boiling hot water for 20 to 30 minutes, until soft. Drain and discard the water when ready.

Preheat the oven to 350°F (175°C, or gas mark 4). Line and lightly grease an 8-inch (20-cm) loaf pan with parchment paper. Set aside.

To make the shortbread: Mix all the ingredients together until a smooth batter forms. Press it evenly into the lined loaf pan in a single layer. Bake it for 11 to 12 minutes, or until cooked. It may still be soft, which is okay. Carefully pop it into the freezer.

To make the caramel filling: Combine all the ingredients in a food processor until smooth. Once the shortbread layer is cooled to handle, drizzle the filling and spread it with the back of a spoon. Pop it into the freezer to set.

To make the topping: Combine the chocolate and oil in a small saucepan over low heat. (Or you can zap in the microwave for 30 seconds.) Melt the chocolate and coconut oil together until you have a smooth chocolate.

Pour the melted chocolate over the filling of your bars and spread it evenly by moving your loaf tin around so it's evenly distributed. Finish with some flaky salt and let it finish setting in the freezer for 5 minutes.

Remove from the freezer and use parchment paper to remove the chocolate bars from the loaf tin. Using a serrated sharp knife, cut 8 pieces out. Serve immediately or store in the fridge or freezer in an airtight container.

Make It AIP

Use tigernut butter in place of tahini. Use ¼ cup (24 g) of carob powder in place of chocolate. Omit vanilla extract or sub vanilla powder or alcohol-free vanilla extract.

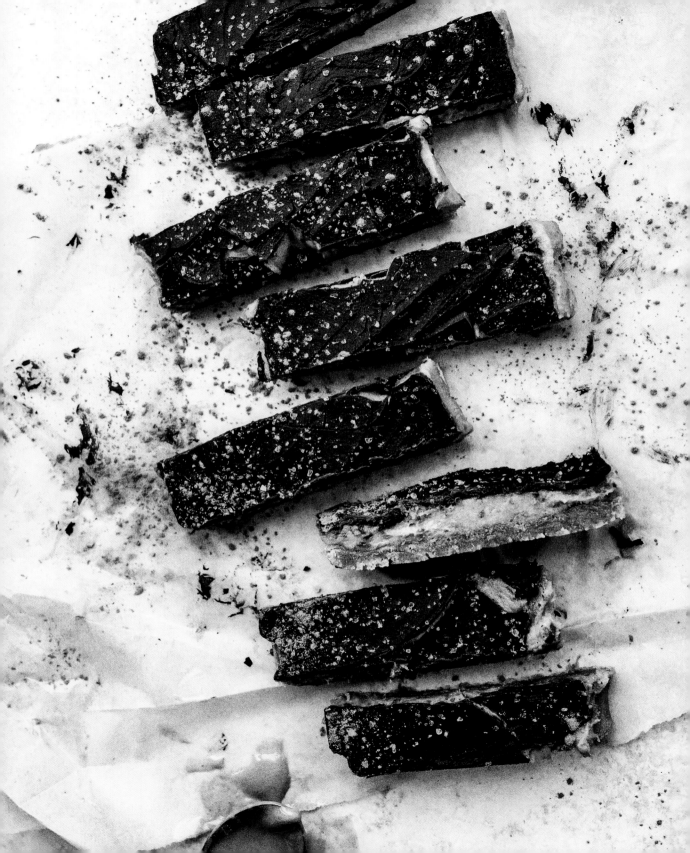

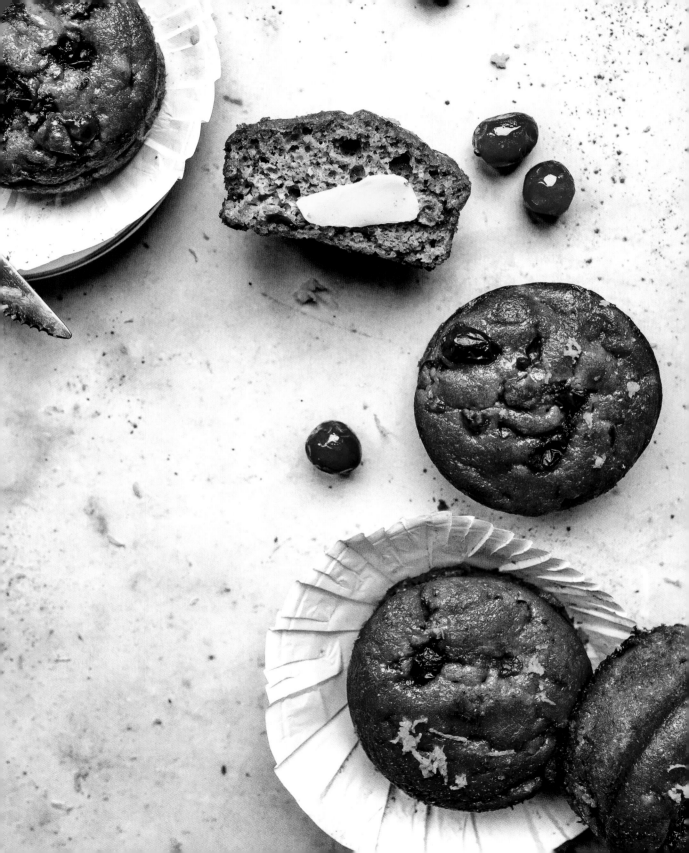

Cranberry Orange Flourless Muffins

The magic of these muffins is from using creamy nut butter and fresh eggs, which combine to form soft, chewy, fluffy muffins. They're only lightly sweetened but so flavorful. For another flavor variation, visit my blog (foodbymars.com) for flourless pumpkin muffins! If you're on AIP, wait to come back to these muffins after reintroducing eggs and nut butter. It's worth the wait!

PREP TIME 10 minutes
COOK TIME 20 minutes
TOTAL TIME 30 minutes
YIELD 12 muffins

¾ cup (184 g) unsweetened applesauce

1 cup (260 g) creamy cashew or almond butter

4–6 tablespoons (60–80 ml) maple syrup, to taste

2 large pasture-raised eggs

1 teaspoon apple cider vinegar

½ teaspoon baking soda

½ teaspoon vanilla extract

½ teaspoon ground cinnamon

1 cup (110 g) cranberries

1 tablespoon (6 g) orange zest

Preheat the oven to 350°F (175°C, or gas mark 4) and place a rack in the middle. Line a 12-cup muffin pan or 24 minis. If you don't have liners, just grease the molds with a little oil.

Mix all ingredients together, except cranberries and orange zest. Combine well until you have a smooth batter.

To a food processor, add cranberries and give it a few quick pulses just to break them up. This helps distribute them more evenly in the batter and makes it tastier! Fold the cranberries and orange zest into the batter with a spatula; reserve a few cranberries for topping. Evenly distribute the batter in your muffin pan. Sprinkle a few cranberries on top of each. Bake for 20 minutes.

Let the muffins cool on a rack for 10 minutes. Serve immediately or store in an airtight container in the fridge for up to 5 days or in the freezer for up to 1 month.

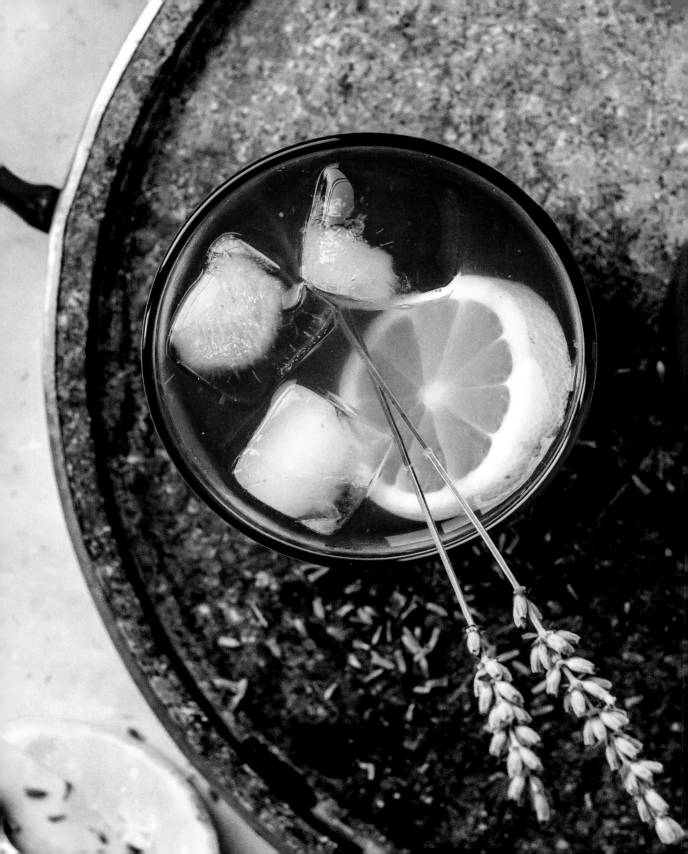

8

DRINKS & TONICS

I invite you to sip on tea, bone broth, or a soothing herbal tonic and make a ritual out of it for yourself and your healing journey. These recipes will give you great options and maybe even expose you to some new flavors and support for your gut! The Rose-Cardamom Marshmallow Root Tea (page 170) is a common after-dinner treat for me, or a Hot Cocoa Bone Broth (page 166) depending on the mood! And to cheers with, grab a soothing and delicious Nettle Tea Mojito Mocktail (page 174).

Hot Cocoa Bone Broth 166

Gold Bone Broth Latte 169

Rose-Cardamom Marshmallow Root Tea 170

Pumpkin Spice Turmeric Latte 173

Nettle Tea Mojito Mocktail 174

Lemon and Ginger Aloe Vera Tonic 176

Rooibos Chai 177

Lavender Lemonade with Aloe 179

Hot Cocoa Bone Broth

Rich, thick hot cocoa gets a gut glow-up with the addition of bone broth! You may be asking "Won't I taste it?" Let me assure you, no! You won't! The mild flavor of chicken broth disappears in the chocolate and spices. The velvety texture makes this an extra decadent and soothing sweet treat. This one has to be skipped on AIP eliminations due to the chocolate: Carob won't be a tasty substitute here. Come back to this once you've been able to reintroduce cacao into your life.

PREP TIME 2 minutes
COOK TIME 10 minutes
TOTAL TIME 12 minutes
YIELD 1 serving

½ cup (117.5 ml) chicken bone broth (page 183)

½ cup (117.5 ml) canned full-fat coconut milk, additive-free

1 ounce (27.5 g) 100% dark chocolate or cacao (or at least 85% cacao)

2 tablespoons (10 g) unsweetened cocoa powder (or cacao powder)

3 tablespoons (45 ml) maple syrup or raw honey

½ teaspoon vanilla extract (alcohol-free for AIP)

½ teaspoon ground cinnamon

¼ teaspoon ground cardamom

¼ teaspoon sea salt

To a small saucepan over medium-low heat, add the broth and coconut milk. Stir well and let it heat up for 2 minutes or so. Add in the chocolate, cacao powder, maple syrup, vanilla, cinnamon, cardamom, and salt while whisking vigorously to break up the chocolate until smooth. Continue to stir until you've brought it all to a low simmer for 3 to 4 minutes. Pour into a mug and serve!

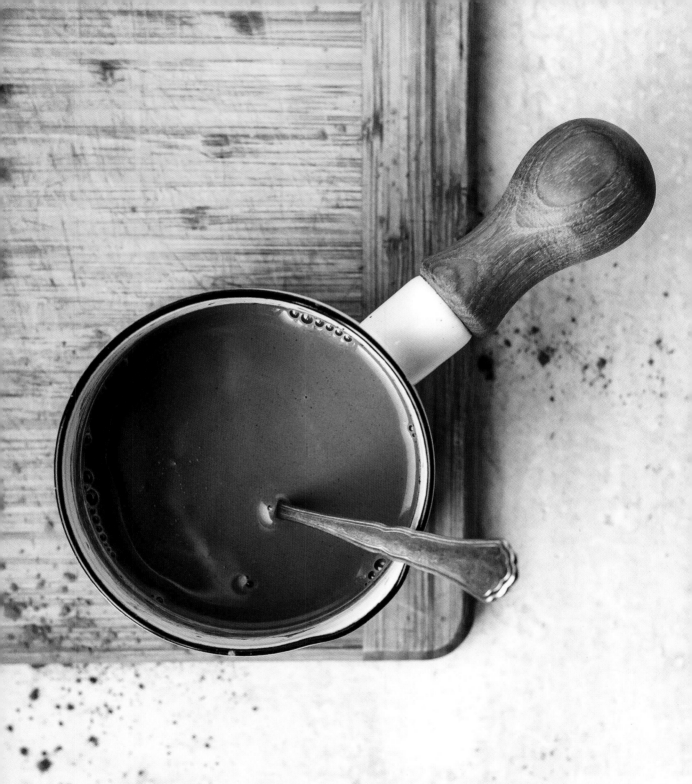

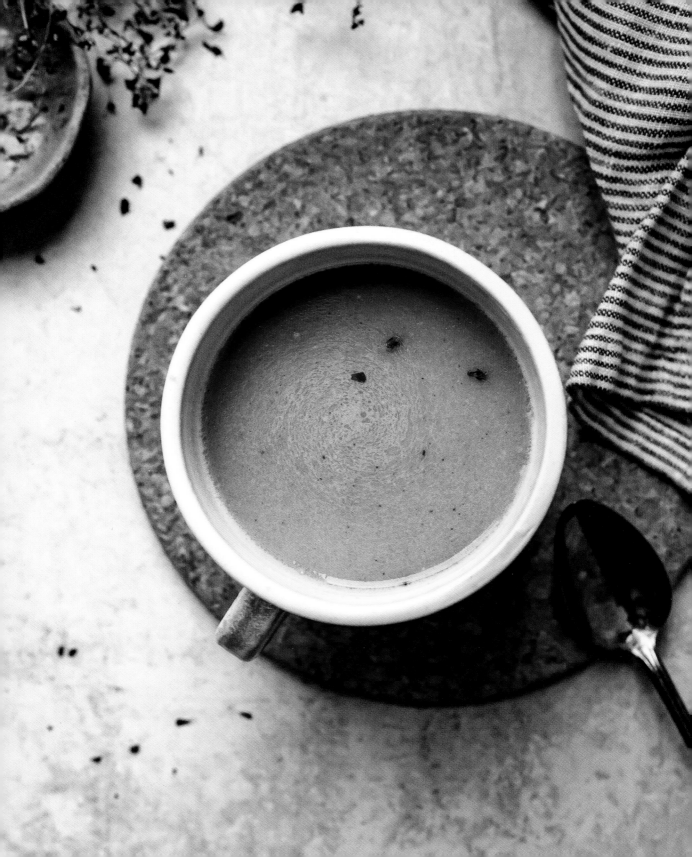

Gold Bone Broth Latte

This soothing latte combines anti-inflammatory turmeric and other spices with fatty coconut milk and healing bone broth to create a smooth and rich drink you'll love to snuggle up with. This is a savory latte, perfect as a snack or morning drink or to accompany any dish. This wonderfully savory drink can be spiced up however you'd like. Try fresh or dried herbs such as ground ginger or garlic!

PREP TIME 2 minutes
COOK TIME 10 minutes
TOTAL TIME 12 minutes
YIELD 2 servings

2 cups (475 ml) bone broth, store-bought or homemade (page 183)

½ cup (120 ml) full-fat coconut milk, additive-free

½ tablespoon (7 g) ghee or grass-fed butter (use coconut or olive oil for AIP)

1 teaspoon ground turmeric

⅛ teaspoon ground cloves

¼ teaspoon black pepper (omit for AIP)

⅛ teaspoon sea salt

1 teaspoon thyme or ½ teaspoon dried thyme (optional)

Combine the broth, coconut milk, ghee, turmeric, cloves, pepper, and salt in a small saucepan over medium. Heat to a simmer for 3 to 4 minutes, stirring to meld flavors. Remove from the heat. Optionally give it one last mix with a hand frother for good measure. Pour into 2 cups and optionally garnish with thyme (if using).

Rose-Cardamom Marshmallow Root Tea

The spicy, floral mix on top of a smooth, comforting tea makes a great midafternoon or postdinner soother for your stomach. In traditional folk practices, marshmallow root tea was given to soothe and moisten mucous membranes of the respiratory, digestive, and urinary tracts. It's very soothing and can be taken in tea form or as a tincture. When I have an upset stomach, nothing soothes it better. Make this in bulk by doubling or tripling the recipe and storing it in an airtight container in the fridge. Marshmallow Root Tea may best be avoided on AIP. See how it feels for you or simply make the rose-cinnamon version.

PREP TIME 2 minutes
COOK TIME 10 minutes
TOTAL TIME 12 minutes
YIELD 2 servings

2 tea bags or 2 tablespoons (4 g) loose marshmallow root tea

2 cups (475 ml) filtered water, boiling

2 tablespoons (6 g) loose-cut dried rosebuds

4 cardamom pods (use 1–2 sticks of cinnamon for AIP)

½ teaspoon of raw honey per cup (optional)

To a teapot with diffuser or a French press, add the tea and boiling water. Set a timer for 5 minutes, and let the tea steep. Add the rosebuds and cardamom pods and steep for 5 minutes (for a total of 10 minutes steep time). Strain the tea and pour into cups. Add sweetener (if using) and serve.

Caution

When taken regularly and medicinally, be sure to drink 1 hour apart from medication as the marshmallow can slow down absorption of the medicine.

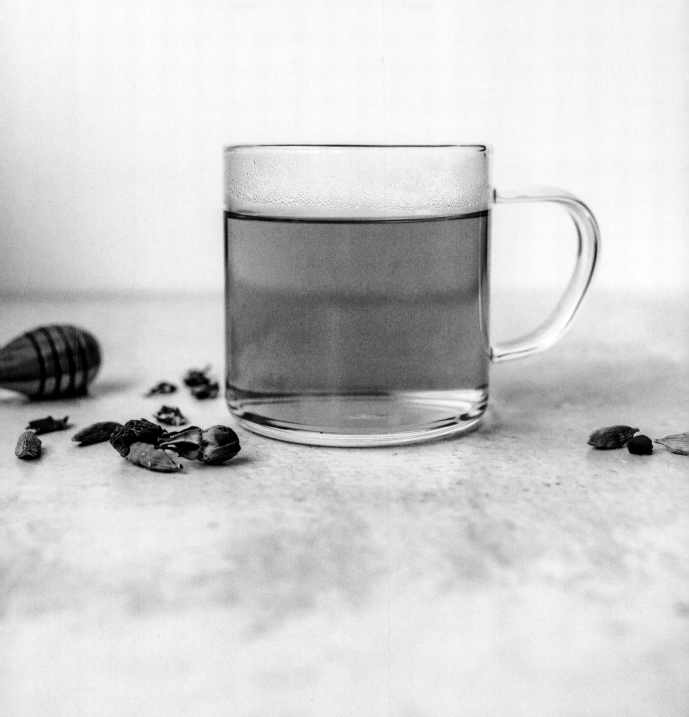

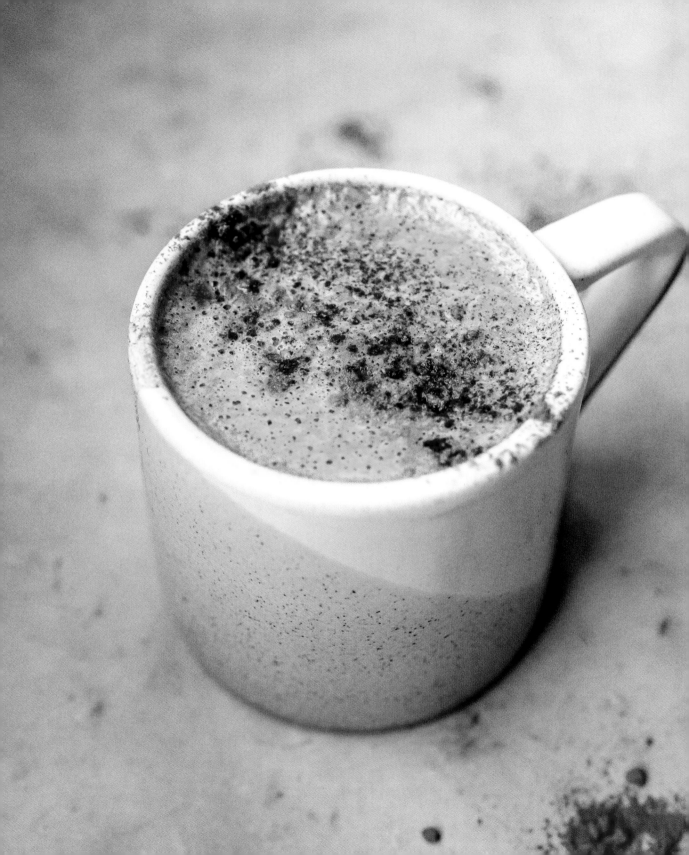

Pumpkin Spice Turmeric Latte

Pumpkin spice latte meets golden turmeric milk for this match-made-in-heaven drink. It's got the "PSL" taste you love, plus anti-inflammatory benefits thanks to the addition of turmeric. This is easy to make and blows that sugar-laden alternative out of the water! Golden milk has ancient Ayurvedic roots and has been used for hundreds of years to aid digestion and as a natural pain reliever. It is commonly used in teas and cooking with a healthy dose of fat and black pepper for absorption.

PREP TIME 5 minutes
COOK TIME 5 minutes
TOTAL TIME 10 minutes
YIELD 1 serving

¾ cup (175 ml) unsweetened nondairy milk (coconut or tigernut milk for AIP)

3 tablespoons (46 g) pumpkin puree

½ teaspoon ground turmeric

1 teaspoon ground cinnamon, plus more for serving

1 teaspoon coconut oil, melted

½ teaspoon vanilla extract (gluten- and alcohol-free for AIP)

¼ teaspoon grated ginger or ½ teaspoon ground

¼ teaspoon ground nutmeg

¼ teaspoon ground clove

⅛ teaspoon ground cardamom (omit for AIP)

⅛ teaspoon black pepper (omit for AIP)

½ teaspoon raw honey or maple syrup (optional)

¼ cup (60 ml) full-fat coconut milk, additive-free

In a small saucepan or butter warmer, add all the ingredients, except the full-fat coconut milk. Whisk over low heat for 5 minutes, until well heated and somewhat combined. The puree should be dissolved; the spices will likely not be.

Transfer the mixture to a blender. Blend on high until you have a thicker, smooth orange-colored milk with spices combined. Pour into a mug.

Steam the coconut milk in a frother or use a hand-held frother. You can also heat it separately, rinse your blender, and blend on high until you have a nice foam. Pour the coconut milk on top of your pumpkin spice turmeric milk. Add a little more cinnamon and serve.

Recipe Tip

To make this iced, simply add all ingredients to a blender without heating it and pour over ice!

Nettle Tea Mojito Mocktail

Reducing or omitting alcohol in the name of gut health doesn't have to leave you empty-handed at a holiday or party when you can make a delicious, soothing nettle tea with zesty mojito flavors from lime and mint. Stinging nettle acts as an antioxidant, antimicrobial, antiulcer, astringent, and analgesic. If you'd like a dose of live cultures with your mojito, substitute the sparkling water with kombucha! Skip this one while on AIP, as phytochemicals in nettle can impact immune function.

PREP TIME 2 minutes
COOK TIME 5 minutes
TOTAL TIME 7 minutes
YIELD 2 servings

2 nettle tea bags

½ teaspoon raw honey

1 lime, halved

½ cup (48 ml) mint leaves, plus more for garnish

1 cup (140 g) crushed ice

½ cup (120 ml) sparkling mineral water or cold filtered water

Brew the tea bags with ½ cup (120 ml) hot water in a cup or teapot according to directions on the package, about 5 minutes. Add ¼ teaspoon of raw honey to each glass and stir to dissolve in the hot water and allow it to cool off for 5 to 10 minutes.

Pour your tea into cocktail glasses. Squeeze half a lime in each glass and stir. Tear mint leaves up by hand to release some of the oils and divide evenly among glasses, muddling with a spoon in the bottom of the glass.

Add crushed ice, and fill the glass with sparkling water. Garnish with whole mint leaves.

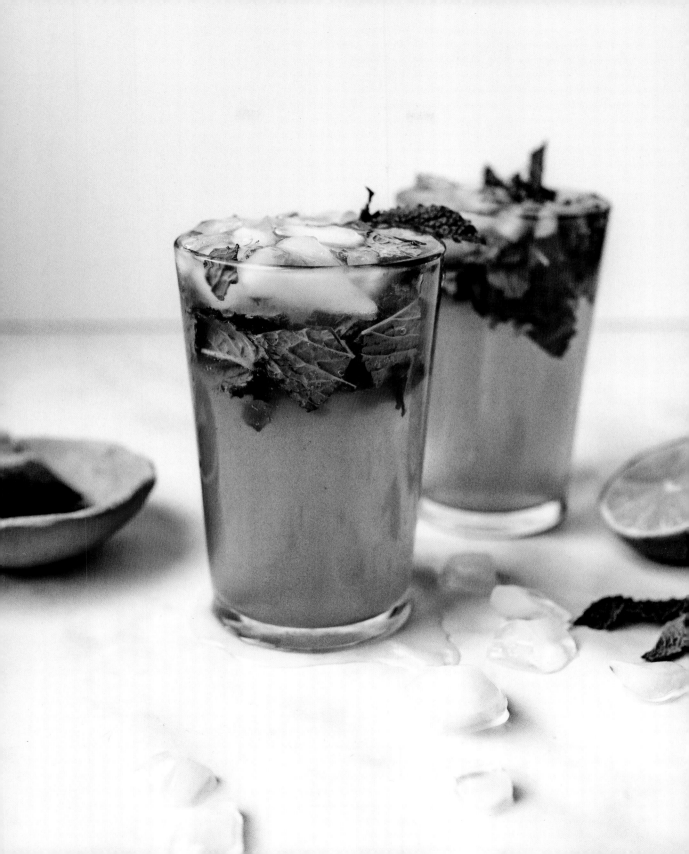

Lemon and Ginger Aloe Vera Tonic

If you're having trouble digesting or are in the middle of a digestive flare-up, whip this tonic up to sip on. It makes a soothing after-meal drink, but is also fabulous to have 15 to 30 minutes before a meal, since it has soothing benefits for the upper GI from the aloe vera juice. The brand of aloe vera juice I use is called Lily of the Desert.

PREP TIME 5 minutes
COOK TIME 5 minutes
TOTAL TIME 10 minutes
YIELD 1 serving

1 cup (235 ml) filtered water, boiled

1 knob (1 inch, or 2.5 cm) of ginger

1 tablespoon (15 ml) fresh lemon juice

1 ounce (28 ml) unsweetened whole leaf aloe vera juice (omit for AIP)

Add boiling water to a large mug with the ginger. Let sit for 5 to 10 minutes. Discard the ginger if you'd like or let it sit at the bottom. Add the lemon juice and aloe vera juice.

You can make this in bulk in a French press and store it in the fridge. Warm up the tonic before serving or add it to room temperature water.

Recipe Tip

Skip the aloe vera on the elimination phase of AIP as it's an immune stimulator, but still enjoy lemon and ginger!

Rooibos Chai

Rooibos (ROY-boss), or red tea, is a delicious caffeine-free herbal tea that's native to South Africa. Rooibos has been used to relieve eczema and allergies and to help babies with colic and insomnia for hundreds of years! More benefits may include soothing an upset stomach, promoting better sleep, and incorporating more antioxidants into your diet. Adding delicious chai spices such as cardamom, cloves, cinnamon, and more make this a warm hug in a mug, without the jitters!

PREP TIME 5 minutes
COOK TIME 10 minutes
TOTAL TIME 15 minutes
YIELD 2 servings

4 cardamom pods (omit for AIP)

4 whole cloves

2 peppercorns (omit for AIP)

1 cinnamon stick

2 star anise (omit for AIP)

½ teaspoon ground ginger

4 teaspoons (2.5 g) loose rooibos tea or the contents of 2 rooibos tea bags

1 cup (235 ml) filtered water

1 cup (235 ml) full-fat additive-free coconut milk, plus more for topping

½ teaspoon vanilla extract (alcohol-free for AIP)

Ground cinnamon (optional)

Using a spoon or mortar and pestle, gently crush the cardamom pods, cloves, peppercorns, cinnamon stick, and star anise. In a saucepan or butter warmer, add all the ingredients, except vanilla and ground cinnamon. Bring to a low simmer over medium heat, stirring occasionally. Let simmer over low heat for 7 to 10 minutes.

Strain out the tea and spices. Mix in the vanilla. You can optionally add heated and frothed coconut milk (¼ cup, or 60 ml, per cup). Garnish with ground cinnamon (if using).

Recipe Tip

Make this iced by storing in an airtight container in the refrigerator for 30 to 60 minutes. Serve over ice.

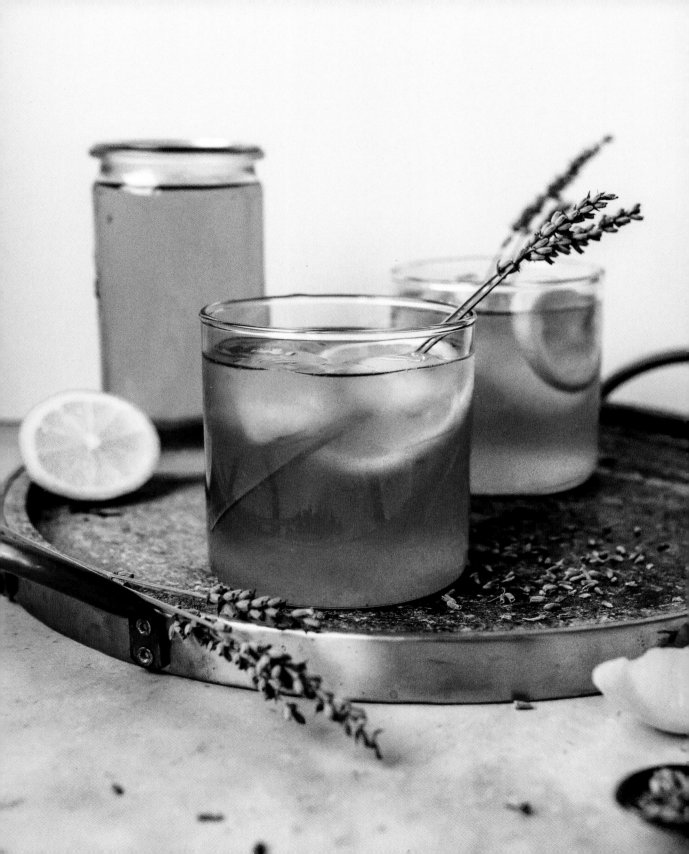

Lavender Lemonade with Aloe

This is a refreshing and delicious midday iced lemonade with soothing upper GI healing benefits from a dose of whole-leaf aloe vera juice! Aloe vera contains several enzymes known to help in the breakdown of sugars and fats. Enjoy this 15 to 30 minutes before a meal to help soothe and prepare for digestion. It's also an effective support to prevent or soothe heartburn and acid reflux symptoms.

PREP TIME 1 to 6 hours

COOK TIME 3 minutes

TOTAL TIME at least 1 hour and 3 minutes

YIELD 1 serving

LAVENDER CONCENTRATE

¼ cup (10 g) culinary lavender

4 cups (940 ml) cold filtered water

LEMONADE

¼ cup (60 ml) unsweetened whole-leaf aloe vera juice (omit for AIP)

1 tablespoon (15 ml) fresh lemon juice

½ teaspoon raw honey

Ice

To make the lavender concentrate: Combine the lavender and water in a 1-quart (1-L) airtight container. Seal and let sit for at least 1 hour and up to 6 hours. Strain and store in the refrigerator.

To make the lemonade: Add the aloe vera juice and lemon juice to a glass. Mix the honey in; if it's thick, you can mix it with 1 teaspoon of hot water and then pour it in. Stir well to combine. Add ¾ cup (175 ml) of lavender concentrate and mix. Fill the rest of your glass with ice, and let sit for 2 minutes to meld.

Store leftover lavender concentrate in the refrigerator for up to 2 weeks. Use it alone as a tea or add it to black tea for a "lavender fog latte" or try it in matcha! It's lightly floral and so delicious; a tiny pinch of sweetener helps round out the flavor even more.

Recipe Tip

Skip the aloe vera on the elimination phase of AIP as it's an immune stimulator, but still enjoy lemon and lavender!

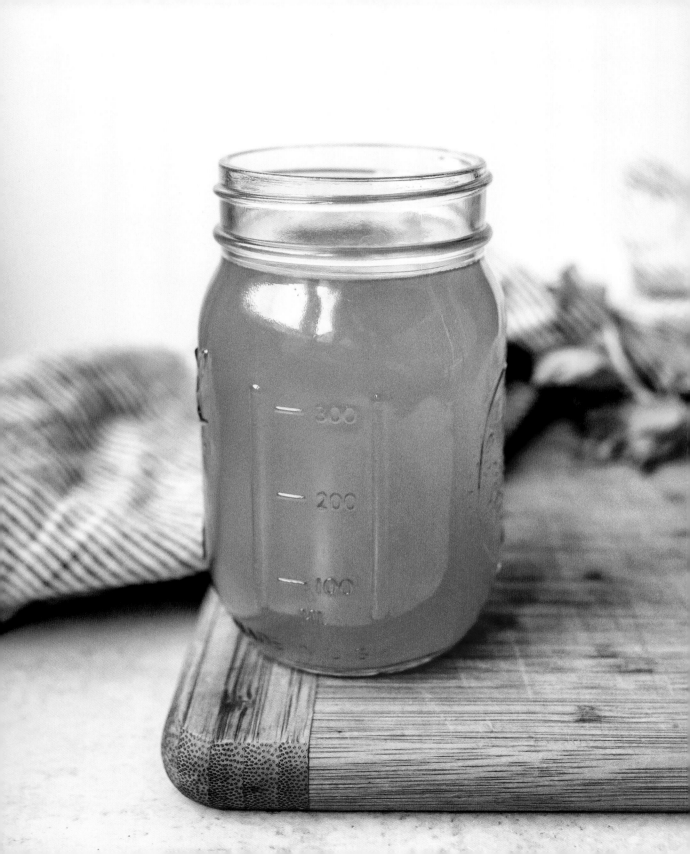

9

STAPLES & CONDIMENTS

Having a few staple recipes in your back pocket means being able to whip up a flavorful, nutrient-dense meal anytime because you've prepared for it! Use the broths for sipping, as cooking liquids, or in soups and sauces. The toppings and other "accessories" are easy ways to elevate your meals in a flash.

Basic Broth 182

Slow Cooker Bone Broth 183

Fermented Coleslaw 184

Instant Pot Coconut Yogurt 187

"Cheese" Sauce 188

Chimichurri 191

Salsa Verde 192

Mango Salsa 193

Mushroom Truffle Pâté 194

Basic Broth

This is my favorite basic broth, and I add in a little more flavor with veggies and aromatics. Get creative with the herbs, vegetables, and aromatics to create different flavor profiles. Try ginger, lemongrass, and fennel for a light, fresh taste in warmer months. Or for a more robust warming taste in the colder months, use rosemary and thyme. Make this in bulk and freeze it for cooking and drinking. If you prefer, make it in a slow cooker or Instant Pot!

PREP TIME 10 minutes
COOK TIME 4 to 6 hours
TOTAL TIME 4 to 6 hours
YIELD 3 to 4 quarts
(2.8 L to 3.8 L)

1 whole (3–4 lb., or 1.4–1.8 kg) free-range organic chicken or turkey

2 chicken feet (optional)

2 large onions, ends cut off and cut into quarters (skin on)

1 head of garlic, cut in half widthwise to expose cloves (skin on)

2 carrots, coarsely chopped

2 celery stalks, coarsely chopped

2 bay leaves

2 tablespoons (28 ml) apple cider or white vinegar (sub lemon juice if you have sensitivities)

Remove the neck, fat glands, and innards from the chicken or turkey cavity. Set the neck aside for the broth, and discard or store the rest for cooking.

To a heavy-bottomed pot, add the bird, chicken feet (if using), neck, and all the veggies and herbs. Add the vinegar and enough filtered water to cover the whole bird; it's okay if it floats up.

Cover and bring to a boil over medium-high heat, then reduce to medium-low and simmer, covered, for 4 to 6 hours. Check occasionally and skim off the scum that rises to the top with a mesh spoon.

Turn off the heat. Gently remove the bird using 2 large spoons, being mindful of the water inside the cavity. Set the bird aside on a cutting board. When cool enough to handle, pick the meat off for later meals and store in an airtight container in the refrigerator for up to 5 days.

Strain the broth through a fine-mesh sieve into another pot or large bowl. Using a ladle or large mug, use a wide-mouth funnel to carefully transfer the broth to airtight containers.

I use 3 to 4 1-quart (946-ml) jars, so I can use it little by little. If freezing, leave 1 to 2 inches (2.5 to 5 cm) of headspace because the liquid expands as it freezes. You can also pour the broth into silicone ice cube trays and store frozen cubes in a freezer bag for convenience.

Store the broth in the refrigerator for up to 7 days. Freeze the broth up to 6 months.

Recipe Tip

Shorter-cooked broths are best to use if bone broth causes a digestive reaction (see page 42 for details). Traditionally, basic broth was used for new mothers in postpartum, infants, the elderly, and those recovering from illness.

Slow Cooker Bone Broth

Your house will smell like a cozy, warm hug as this simmers, and the gut-healing benefits are incredible. You can use this same cooking method on the stovetop in a large stockpot or Dutch oven, but I love using a slow cooker so it's out of the way! Use this broth for sipping, cooking, and more. (See photo on page 180.)

PREP TIME 10 minutes
COOK TIME 24 hours
TOTAL TIME 1 day
YIELD about 4 quarts (3.8 L)

4 pounds (1.8 kg) cooked chicken bones

2 chicken feet (optional)

¼ cup (60 ml) apple cider vinegar (or lemon juice)

2 large onions, ends cut off and cut into quarters (skin left on)

1 garlic head, cut in half widthwise to expose cloves (skin left on)

2 carrots, coarsely chopped

2 celery stalks, coarsely chopped

2 bay leaves

To a slow cooker, add the bones, chicken feet (if using), vinegar, vegetables, and bay leaves. Fill with just enough filtered water to cover the top of the bones. Cover and set your slow cooker for at least 24 hours over low heat to simmer.

When complete, carefully remove the bones and veggies with tongs or large utensils. Discard.

Strain the broth through a fine-mesh sieve into another pot or large bowl, and using a ladle or large mug, carefully transfer the broth into airtight containers. Use a wide-mouth funnel to keep it tidy!

I recommend splitting the broth up into 1-quart (1-L) mason jars so you may use it little by little. When freezing in glass jars, leave 1 to 2 inches empty at the top because the liquid will expand as it freezes. Another option for freezing is to pour broth into silicone ice cube trays and store frozen cubes in a jar or freezer bag for convenience.

Store the broth in the refrigerator for up to 7 days and freeze the broth for up to 6 months. Bone broth may become gelatinous as it cools, and you may also notice a layer of fat at the top of your broth. If it's thick, spoon that out and save it separately in the fridge and use it as cooking fat (*schmaltz*).

To make this on the stovetop, follow the same instructions; you'll just be a little more careful and watchful! To make this in an Instant Pot, set it to high pressure for 120 minutes and allow the pressure to naturally release for at least 30 minutes.

Fermented Coleslaw

Fermented vegetables are easy to make, and the possibilities are endless. I call this "fermented coleslaw" because I'm using cabbage and carrots found in coleslaw mixes. I spice it up with red onion and oregano—a nod to a traditional fermented dish called *curtido* that usually includes jalapeños. A forkful of this stuff a day is a natural, nutrient-dense way to get your probiotics through food. The equipment needed is inexpensive and will make it a heck of a lot easier to do this—be prepared so it's no-fuss and turns out delicious!

PREP TIME 10 minutes
FERMENT TIME 3 to 10 days
TOTAL TIME up to 10 days
YIELD about 12 ounces (340 g)

FERMENTED COLESLAW
2 pounds (907 g) cabbage (from 1 medium head)

1 cup (110 g) carrots, shredded or grated

1 small red onion or ½ large, sliced thinly

½ tablespoon (2 g) dried oregano

4 teaspoons (22 g) sea salt

EQUIPMENT
Glass jar (mason jars work well)

A small weight (e.g., a fermentation weight) to fit inside the jar or one smaller jar that fits inside the larger one (e.g., a jelly jar) that you can fill with dry beans, rocks, or water to weigh the vegetables down and ensure they stay submerged under water

Airlock (recommended)

Mandoline (or chef's knife) and cutting board

Remove the outermost leaves from your cabbage and any that are bruised or damaged, then slice it in half crosswise. Remove the core, then slice the cabbage thinly using a mandolin, food processor, or sharp chef's knife (no wider than ⅛ inch thick).

In a large mixing bowl, mix the cabbage, carrots, onion, oregano, and salt together. Let it rest for 20 minutes, or until the cabbage softens and releases some juice. Massage and squeeze the vegetables with your hands to soften it and help it to release more juice.

When the cabbage has become limp and has released enough juice so the vegetables are nearly submerged, transfer it all to your jar. Pack the vegetables very tightly into your jar, using a wooden spoon, so the vegetables continue to release liquid and no air bubbles remain.

Continue packing the mixture into the container until it is completely submerged by its liquid. Place a weight over the mixture, then seal the jar with your airlock (or tightly seal the mason jar).

Allow the mixture to ferment at room temperature and away from direct sunlight or heat for at least 5 days and up to 1 month, or until done to your liking. You can taste it after 5 days to check in on it and re-seal. If you see any mold inside the jar, discard the whole batch and be cautious to use clean hands and clean utensils after handling it.

Once the fermented coleslaw tastes good to you, transfer it to the fridge, where it will keep at least 6 months and up to 1 year if it's submerged in the liquid.

Recipe Tips

Always use clean hands and clean utensils whenever handling the ferment.

Vegetables will ferment quicker in hotter months or a hotter climate, so keep an eye on it.

Discard the batch if you find any mold.

Noticing air bubbles as it ferments is normal and expected.

Using a weight is necessary to keep the vegetables submerged as it ferments.

If you need to use more liquid and it's not releasing enough on its own in the beginning preparation stage, you can create a brine with 1 teaspoon salt per 1 cup (235 ml) of filtered water.

Fermentation is an anaerobic process, so it's best when there's limited air flow. An airlock is best; otherwise you need to make sure it's tightly sealed or mold can occur. You can add a cheesecloth to the top of your jar and then seal it.

You'll know when the fermentation process is happening after your taste test. It should taste pleasantly sour and have a slightly similar aroma to vinegar.

Once you place the ferment in the fridge, the fermentation process will stop.

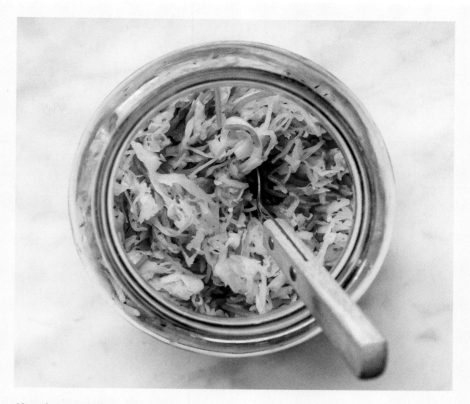

Alter the seasonings to taste or even add jalapeño slices to make it a true Salvadorian *curtido*.

The salt-to-cabbage ratio is important: Salt feeds the good bacteria and keeps bad bacteria and mold at bay. It also aids in the crispness of the vegetables so it's not a mushy mess. Salt is used for both safety and texture!
The rule of thumb is: for every 1 pound of cabbage you use, add 1½ to 2 teaspoons of salt. A good fine sea salt, Celtic sea salt, or similar makes a great mineral-rich salt to use.

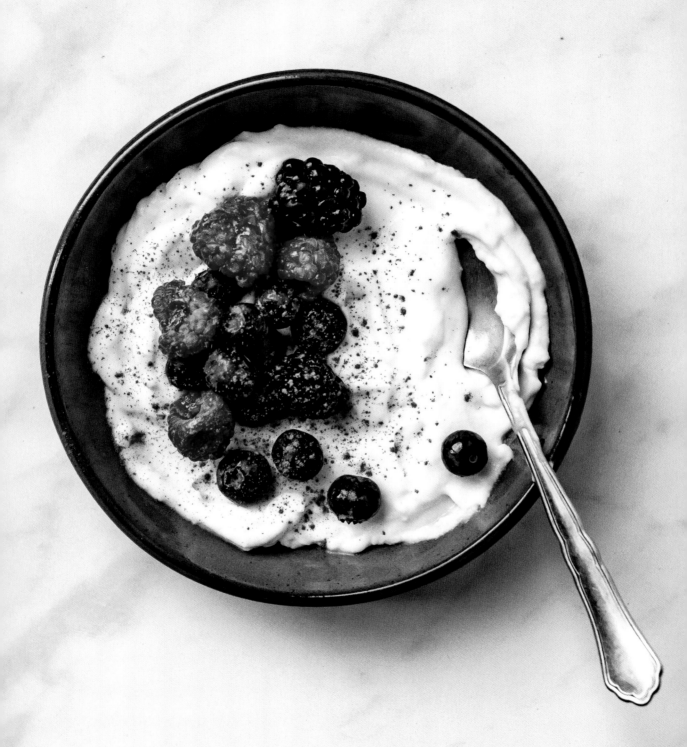

Instant Pot Coconut Yogurt

Using an electric pressure cooker (Instant Pot) is one of the easiest ways to make coconut yogurt at home with the least fuss or stress! It's delicious, creamy, and you can customize it to your own taste and preferences with sweetness, tanginess, and thickness.

PREP TIME 10 minutes
FERMENT TIME 12+ hours
TOTAL TIME 12+ hours
YIELD about 27 ounces (765 g)

COCONUT YOGURT

2 cans (13.5 ounces, or 383 g) full-fat additive-free coconut milk (I use Native Harvest.)

1 tablespoon (15 ml) maple syrup

2 teaspoons (6 g) grass-fed gelatin

1 package (0.06-ounce) dairy-free yogurt starter culture (I use Cultures for Health) or 1–2 lactobacillus-based probiotic capsule(s), 15 to 20 billion PFU (or CFU)

EQUIPMENT

Instant Pot with yogurt setting

Kitchen thermometer

Jars

Pour the coconut milk and maple syrup into the Instant Pot. Whisk well to combine. Leave the lid off and press the "Yogurt" button and adjust the setting until it reads "boil" on the digital face. Let it run and heat up while whisking occasionally.

Once the Instant Pot beeps, it will start to cool. Allow it to cool off until it's 110°F (43°C). This can take around 1 hour; just keep an eye on it.

Once the temperature reaches 110°F (43°C) degrees, whisk in the gelatin well and stir. Once that's combined, add the culture (from the yogurt starter or by opening the probiotic capsules). Whisk again, very well.

Close the lid on the Instant Pot and press the "Yogurt" button. Adjust the time to at least 12 hours for a good amount of tang and creaminess. Once it's done fermenting, taste it. If you'd like it tangier, you can add more time (not going above 36 hours in total).

Once it's done to your liking, pour the mixture into airtight containers. Cool for at least 2 hours; it will continue to thicken in the fridge. Divide among smaller mason jars so it cools faster and is easier to grab and go.

Serve as desired with berries and other toppings, or use in cooking. Keep it stored in the refrigerator in airtight containers for up to 10 days.

Recipe Tips

I prefer using the yogurt culture starter. If you use capsules, opt for a non-soil-based probiotic capsule for a better taste. You can save 4 tablespoons (60 ml) of your finished yogurt and use it in your next batch as the starter culture using this same recipe. That way, you just need to buy the starter once and can continue using your last batch as a new starter.

Choose maple syrup over honey, which has its own bacteria. I start with just 1 tablespoon if I want to use it in savory dishes and can add more if I'd like it to be sweet later. Sweeten it more, if you prefer.

"Cheese" Sauce

This creamy, nut-free, AIP-friendly cheese sauce is a reader fave! Even the picky cheese-loving eaters will devour it. I love it for a simple "nachos" dish with ground meat hash (page 94) and some sweet potato or plantain chips!

PREP TIME 10 minutes
COOK TIME 5 minutes
TOTAL TIME 15 minutes
YIELD 2 cups (486 g)

2 cups (248 g) steamed cauliflower

1 cup (240 g) coconut cream, additive-free

2 tablespoons (10 g) nutritional yeast

¼ cup (60 ml) water

2 tablespoons (18 g) arrowroot

½ tablespoon (8 ml) lemon juice or apple cider vinegar

½ teaspoon sea salt

¼ teaspoon garlic powder

Add all ingredients to a high-speed blender and blend on high until well combined. Use immediately or store in an airtight container in the refrigerator for up to 5 days or frozen in small jars for up to 1 month. Defrost as needed in a hot water bath to pour on your favorite dishes.

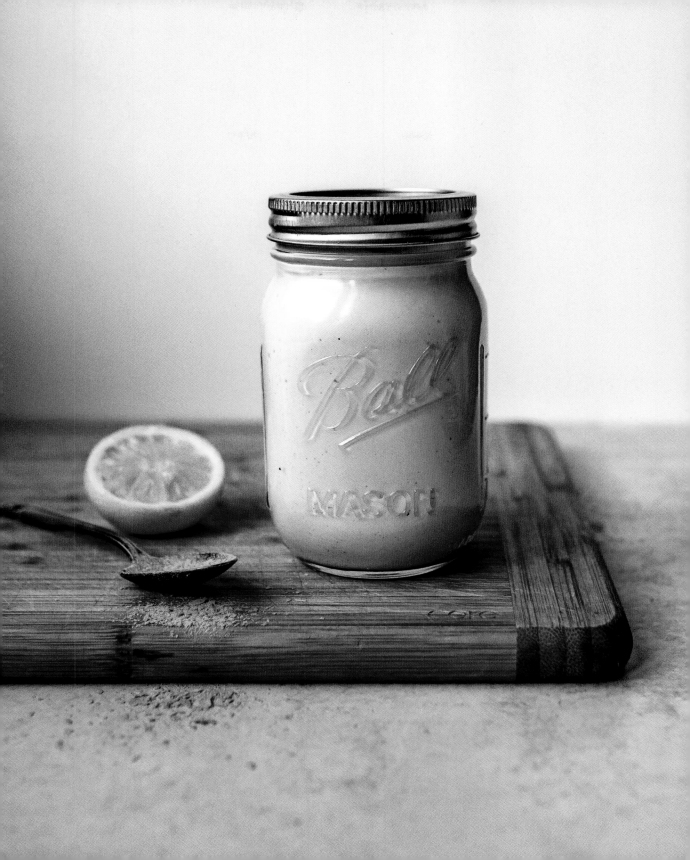

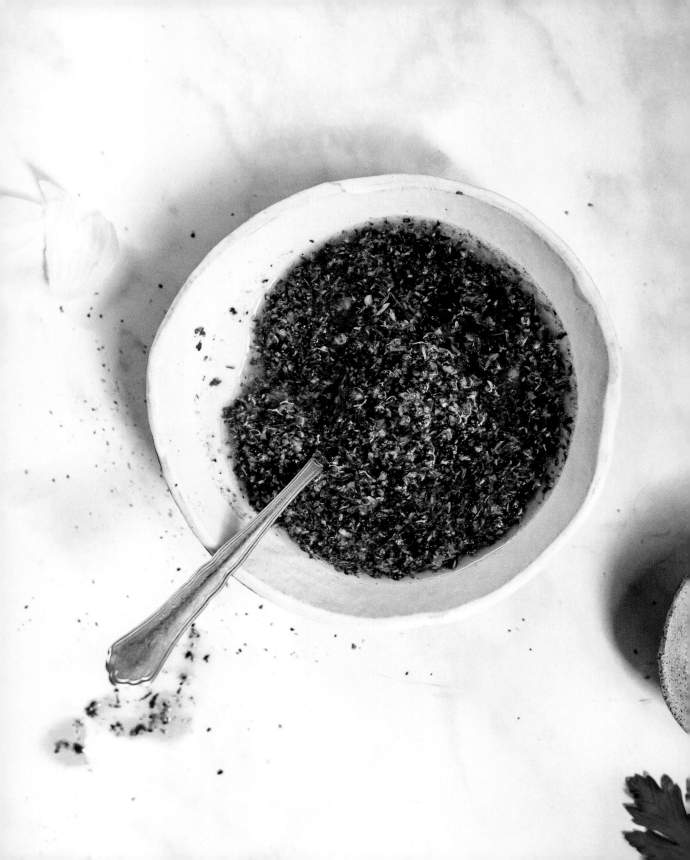

Chimichurri

This gorgeous green flavor-bomb of a sauce is great on protein, veggies, and more. It's especially delicious paired with red meat, but you'll love it so much, you may find yourself slathering it on all things, just as I do. Parsley may assist the kidneys and digestive system and help to relieve gastrointestinal symptoms.

PREP TIME 5 minutes
COOK TIME 5 minutes
TOTAL TIME 10 minutes
YIELD ½ cup (120 g)

¼ cup (15 g) flat-leaf Italian parsley

1 tablespoon (9 g) capers

1 tablespoon (15 ml) red wine vinegar

1 tablespoon (3 g) dried oregano

1 tablespoon (4 g) red pepper flakes (omit for AIP)

4 cloves garlic, minced

¼ teaspoon sea salt

½ cup (118 ml) extra-virgin olive oil

Add all ingredients, except the oil, to a food processor. Mix until well combined.

Add the oil and mix again to form your sauce. Season to taste. Store in the fridge for 5 to 6 days in an airtight container, or for up to 1 month in the freezer. Freeze this versatile sauce in ice cube trays and store away in a freezer bag. Simply grab a cube to add a sauce to any savory dish, or drop it into your broth for soups and stocks!

Salsa Verde

Green sauces are the best! This one gives an instant flavor burst to any dish. Cilantro (and coriander) can help prevent and relieve indigestion and heartburn symptoms, and it stimulates the release of digestive enzymes, which helps to assimilate the nutrients and aid in stronger digestion.

PREP TIME 5 minutes
COOK TIME 5 minutes
TOTAL TIME 10 minutes
YIELD ½ cup (120 g)

⅓ cup (5 g) cilantro, stems removed

⅓ cup (13 g) basil, stems removed

1 clove garlic, minced

¼ cup (40 g) chopped red onion

Juice of ½ lemon

¼ teaspoon sea salt

1–2 teaspoons extra-virgin olive oil as desired

Add all the ingredients, except the oil, to a food processor. Mix until well combined. Add the oil and mix again to form your sauce. Taste and season as necessary!

Serve as a sauce, topping, or dip. Store in the fridge for 5 to 6 days in an airtight container, or for up to 1 month in the freezer. Freeze in ice cube trays and grab a cube to make a sauce or flavor your broth for soups and stocks.

Mango Salsa

Mango is one of my favorite additions to a sauce! It's packed with sweetness and tartness, and it adds great texture. This pairs well with any protein, or serve it on a platter with your favorite veggies or Paleo-friendly chips for a party.

PREP TIME 5 minutes
COOK TIME 5 minutes
TOTAL TIME 10 minutes
YIELD about ½ to ⅓ cup (129.5 g)

1 mango, chopped

¼ cup (40 g) chopped red onion

⅓ heaping cup (5 g) chopped cilantro

Juice of 1 lime

¼ teaspoon sea salt, plus more to taste

Add the mango, onion, cilantro, lime juice, and salt to a food processor. Pulse until the salsa forms. Season to taste with additional salt.

Serve as a sauce or dip, and store in the refrigerator for up to 5 days in an airtight container.

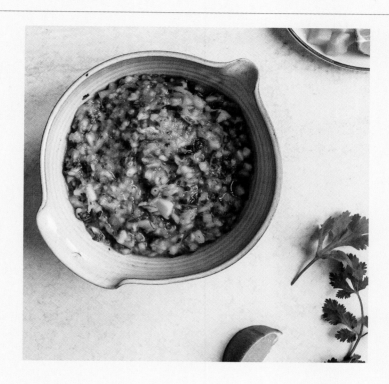

Recipe Tip

Mango makes a fabulous substitute for tomatoes. To make a mango guacamole, add some diced avocado. Mash by hand for a chunkier guac, or pulse in the food processor for a smooth mango guac.

Mushroom Truffle Pâté

If eating liver or other offal turns you off, give pâté a chance! This French "spread" is made of liver, herbs, and good fat. We are flavoring it up with mushrooms and truffle oil. Serve with vegetables such as raw carrots, celery, or endive; sweet potato toast; Paleo-friendly crackers; plantain or sweet potato chips; or simply alone on a side or topping.

PREP TIME 10 minutes
COOK TIME 15 minutes plus 2 to 3 hours to chill
TOTAL TIME 2 to 3 hours
YIELD 8 servings

1 pound (454 g) chicken liver

¼ cup (52 g) duck fat or lard (for AIP), or ghee

2 medium shallots

8 ounces (225 g) cremini or button mushrooms, sliced

2 cloves garlic

1 teaspoon dried thyme

1 tablespoon (2 g) chopped rosemary or 1 teaspoon dried rosemary

¼ teaspoon sea salt

2 tablespoons (28 ml) balsamic vinegar

2 teaspoons (10 ml) white truffle oil, or more to taste (additive free, real truffles and olive oil only)

½ cup (120 ml) coconut cream, additive-free

Coarse sea salt, extra-virgin olive oil, and herbs, to taste

Trim the chicken liver pieces and discard any fatty, stringy pieces. Rinse and drain all the pieces. Set aside.

To a skillet over medium heat, add your fat. Once hot, add the shallots, stirring occasionally for 2 to 3 minutes, until they're softened. Add the mushrooms and garlic. Cook and stir for 4 to 5 minutes, or until the mushrooms are softened.

Add the chicken liver and season everything with thyme, rosemary, and salt. Stir well to combine and cook for 7 to 8 minutes, or until the liver is cooked through. Add the balsamic vinegar, stirring, and let it caramelize on the liver for 2 to 3 minutes. Break up the liver a bit with a wooden spoon to make sure it's fully cooked inside.

Once the liver is fully cooked and the vinegar has been absorbed, turn off the heat and transfer the mixture to a food processor or high-speed blender. Add the truffle oil and coconut cream. Blend until smooth. Taste and adjust seasonings as needed.

Spoon out the mixture into a small baking dish or ramekins, pressing it into the dish firmly (no air bubbles). Cover with plastic wrap or parchment paper, touching the mixture. If your dish has a lid, add that on top or use aluminum foil for more reinforcement (and to keep it from overpowering the fridge). Refrigerate for at least 3 hours, until chilled. Store in an airtight container refrigerated for up to 5 days.

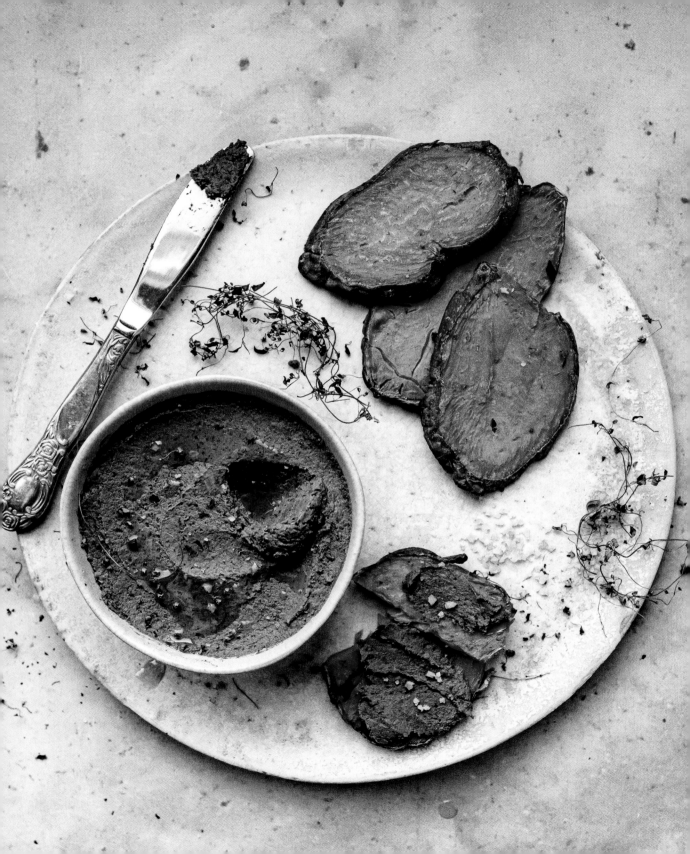

10

2-WEEK GUT REFRESH MEAL PLAN

This meal plan immerses you in your gut-healthy lifestyle! Approach it openly and lovingly. It is not a quick fix, though you should feel relief. It's meant to be a tool for you to expand on with your bio-individuality in mind. To help support your refresh, review the everyday practices detailed in chapter 2 (page 23) and choose a strategy (or two!) that you can easily integrate into your plan. Maybe you can focus on eating mindfully or managing stress, or maybe you want to prioritize adding variety to your diet. Every small step adds up!

Keep a food journal with you to jot down anything you learn about your body. (Go to foodbymars.com/book-guide for a food/mood journal to print.) At the end of two weeks, assess where you are. If you'd love to continue all or some elements you tried, go for it! Remember, this is a lifestyle you are building and learning from.

Daily Practices

Begin each day with at least 8 ounces (235 ml) of room temperature lemon water (half of a lemon squeezed into your water).

Keep hydrated between meals with room temperature or even warm water, which is optimal for digestion.

Enjoy 1 to 3 cups (235 to 705 ml) of bone broth between meals or with a meal.

Optional: Try a forkful of a fermented food, such as the Fermented Coleslaw (page 184) or sauerkraut, with one of your meals. (If this gives you a digestive reaction, reduce it to just a few times a week or skip it and come back to it after you've done more healing.) You can also try the Instant Pot Coconut Yogurt (page 187), and see what feels best for you and in what quantities!

Pay Attention to How You Eat

The food choices you make matter, but one of the simplest ways to help your digestion is to change *how* you eat. Put yourself in a parasympathetic state and let "rest and digest" set you up for success!

→ Before starting your meal, sit and take at least three to five deep belly breaths.

→ Don't rush through your meals. Take your time, relax, and eat slowly.

→ Practice mindful eating by being present, minimizing distractions, and focusing on the food in front of you (page 24).

→ Savor your meal and chew all food very well.

Helpful Tips

This meal plan serves four. If you are cooking for fewer people, use up leftovers on the weekends or freeze them for later, or divide the recipes in half. If cooking for more people, simply multiply the servings.

If you have chronic upper GI issues, such as reflux or heartburn, try the Lemon and Ginger Aloe Vera Tonic (page 176) 15 minutes before your last or heaviest meal.

For chronic constipation or even diarrhea, try the Rose-Cardamom Marshmallow Root Tea (page 170).

If you are often bloated by the end of meals, try adding in 1 teaspoon of apple cider vinegar to your water 15 minutes before meals to help boost your HCl (stomach acid), and remember to eat mindfully.

If you're new to drinking bone broth, start with 1 cup per day and work your way up. If bone broth gives you a digestive reaction, sub with the Basic Broth recipe (page 182) until you've done more healing. It may take some time for you to be able to handle the high concentration of amino acids found in the bone broth. You can also dilute the bone broth with filtered water (try a 1:1 ratio).

The dessert recipes in this cookbook are low on natural sweeteners and generally gut-friendly in moderation. Enjoy them mindfully and keep it balanced (i.e., one serving/day). If you feel you need a total break from sweets, go without them or stick with only whole fruits. Too much snacking will deter from your progress, so just be honest and kind to yourself.

A note on AIP: If you are trying the AIP versions, be sure to plan ahead for reintroductions. This will help to set you up for success. There are more resources for how to do this on foodbymars.com/book-guide.

WEEK 1

Paleo/AIP-Friendly Gut Refresh Menu

	BREAKFAST	LUNCH	DINNER
MONDAY	Meat Hash with Kale and Cabbage (page 94) with 1 cup bone broth (page 183)	Chicken Zoodle Soup (page 60)	Chicken, Bacon, Brussels Sprouts, and Squash Skillet (page 84) with 1 cup bone broth (page 183)
TUESDAY	Chicken Zoodle Soup (page 60)	Tropical Shrimp Salad (page 144) with 1 cup bone broth (page 183)	Rib Eye Steak with Chimichurri (page 97) with Rosemary Parsnip Puree (page 137) with 1 cup bone broth (page 183)
WEDNESDAY	Meat Hash with Kale and Cabbage (page 94) with mixed greens and 1 cup bone broth (page 183)	Creamy Ginger, Pear, and Butternut Squash Soup (option to add shredded chicken) (page 64)	Crispy Golden Salmon (page 92) with Veggie Confetti Rice (page 133) and 1 cup bone broth (page 183)
THURSDAY	Chicken Zoodle Soup (page 60)	Rib Eye Steak with Chimichurri (page 97) with 1 cup bone broth (page 183)	Tropical Shrimp Salad (page 144) with 1 cup bone broth (page 183)
FRIDAY	Meat Hash with Kale and Cabbage (page 94) with mixed greens and 1 cup bone broth (page 183)	Creamy Ginger, Pear, and Butternut Squash Soup (option to add shredded chicken) (page 64)	Crispy Golden Salmon (page 92) with Veggie Confetti Rice (page 133) and 1 cup bone broth (page 183)

WEEK 2

Paleo/AIP-Friendly Gut Refresh Menu

	BREAKFAST	LUNCH	DINNER
MONDAY	Smoked Salmon Salad with Jammy Eggs (page 148) with mixed greens and 1 cup bone broth (page 183)	Mushroom and Cauliflower Rice Soup with Chicken (page 71)	Teriyaki Salmon and Bok Choy (page 102) with 1 cup bone broth (page 183)
TUESDAY	Italian Wedding Soup (page 63)	Chicken Marbella (page 83) with Crispy Baked Sweet Potato Fries (page 122) and 1 cup bone broth (page 183)	Shrimp and Broccoli (page 103) with 1 cup bone broth (page 183)
WEDNESDAY	Smoked Salmon Salad with Jammy Eggs (page 148) with mixed greens and 1 cup bone broth (page 183)	Italian Wedding Soup (page 63)	Teriyaki Salmon and Bok Choy (page 102) with 1 cup bone broth (page 183)
THURSDAY	Italian Wedding Soup (page 63)	Chicken Marbella (page 83) with Crispy Baked Sweet Potato Fries (page 122) and 1 cup bone broth (page 183)	Mushroom and Cauliflower Rice Soup with Chicken (page 71)
FRIDAY	Smoked Salmon Salad with Jammy Eggs (page 148) with mixed greens and 1 cup bone broth (page 183)	Mushroom and Cauliflower Rice Soup with Chicken (page 71)	Shrimp and Broccoli (page 103) with 1 cup bone broth (page 183)

ABOUT THE AUTHOR

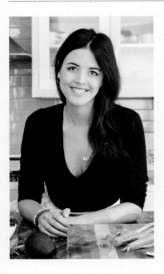

Alison Marras shares delicious gut-loving Paleo and AIP-friendly recipes and wellness tips over at www.foodbymars.com. She believes a healing journey with real food can be a stress-free lifestyle, filled with joy and flavor, and she is dedicated to enabling her audience to take control of their health. Living with Hashimoto's autoimmune disease and PCOS, Alison began her food blog after realizing the importance of food as medicine in helping her heal and in keeping symptoms under control. She combined her love of cooking and mindfulness practices with her health journey in creating helpful content everyone can enjoy! Her career in holistic nutrition and wellness has propelled her to educate, create resources and meal plans, and foster a vibrant community of people committed to healing their bodies with food and lifestyle, joyfully.

To connect and follow along, visit Alison on social media @foodbymars and sign up for her blog newsletter on foodbymars.com!

ACKNOWLEDGMENTS

To my entire family, thank you for helping me make this book come to life. I couldn't have done it without you.

Special shout-outs to:

My husband, for always washing dishes and keeping the kitchen organized after I made it look like a hurricane passed through it. For always believing me and making me feel invincible.

My mom, *abuela*, and mother-in-law, for taking my random calls asking for family recipes scribbled on index cards or imprinted in memory so I could make them Paleo-friendly. And my sister, for the extra babysitting duty and attempting to get me to use my dishwasher more as opposed to hand-washing (working on it, Sis!).

My dear friends, for recipe testing sporadically and sharing your delish food photos and feedback with me!

My daughter, for inspiring me to be more mindful and present, to practice what I preach, and to be a role model to her when following her own passions in life.

To you . . . my amazing readers, clients, friends, and community, for letting me do what I love, for supporting me and cheering me on, and for sharing your food photos and stories with me. You'll never know how much it blesses me!

To my colleagues in the food blogging and nutrition/wellness universe, who inspire me daily with their creativity and mission-driven work.

Lastly, to Jill, Jenna, and Heather—my amazing team in publishing this book. It's been an honor and pleasure to have your support and guidance through this process. Thank you for your passion and grace.

RESOURCES & REFERENCES

While writing this book, I referred to the comprehensive sources listed below for data and research on digestion, supporting gut health with food as medicine, and the Paleo/AIP diets. If you are interested in learning more on these topics, I invite you to explore them further!

Websites

Nutritional Therapy Association Blog and Curriculum: nutritionaltherapy.com

Healthline: healthline.com

Dr. Axe Blog: draxe.com

The Institute for Functional Medicine: ifm.org

Nourished Kitchen Blog: nourishedkitchen.com

Autoimmune Wellness Blog: autoimmunewellness.com

The Paleo Mom by Dr. Sarah Ballantyne: thepaleomom.com

Dr. Datis Kharrazian Blog: drknews.com

Phoenix Helix Blog: phoenixhelix.com

Books and Articles

Alt, Angie, and Mickey Trescott. *The Autoimmune Wellness Handbook: A DIY Guide to Living Well with Chronic Illness.* Rodale Books, 2016.

Ballantyne, Sarah. *Paleo Principles: The Science Behind the Paleo Template, Step-by-Step Guides, Meal Plans, and 200+ Healthy & Delicious Recipes for Real Life.* Victory Belt Publishing, 2017.

Breit, Sigrid, et al. "Vagus Nerve as Modulator of the Brain-Gut Axis in Psychiatric and Inflammatory Disorders." *Frontiers in Psychiatry.* 9, 44, March 13, 2018.

Campbell-McBride, Natasha. *Gut and Psychology Syndrome: Natural Treatment for Autism, Dyspraxia, A.D.D., Dyslexia, A.D.H.D., Depression, Schizophrenia.* Medinform Publishing, 2018.

Mayer, Emeran, MD. *The Mind-Gut Connection: How the Hidden Conversation Within Our Bodies Impacts Our Mood, Our Choices, and Our Overall Health. Blackstone Audio, Inc.* Harper Wave, 2018.

McGruther, Jennifer. *Broth and Stock from the Nourished Kitchen: Wholesome Master Recipes for Bone, Vegetable, and Seafood Broths and Meals to Make with Them.* Ten Speed Press, 2016.

Morrell, Sally Fallon, and Kaayla T. Daniel, Ph.D., CCN. *Nourishing Broth: An Old-Fashioned Remedy for the Modern World.* Grand Central Life and Style, 2014.

Visit foodbymars.com/book-guide to get grocery list printouts, recommended brands, and more resources for easier, cost-effective shopping.

SHOPPING LISTS

Paleo and AIP-Friendly Pantry Staples

⊘ = to be excluded on the AIP elimination phase

Condiments/Sauces

Apple cider vinegar

Balsamic vinegar

Capers

Olives

Mayo (made with extra-virgin olive oil or avocado oil, Paleo-friendly) ⊘

Fish sauce with safe ingredients

Nutritional yeast

White wine vinegar

Coconut aminos (as a soy sauce substitute)

Tomato paste ⊘

Red wine vinegar

Paleo-friendly ketchup or AIP-friendly beet ketchup

Paleo- or AIP-friendly barbecue sauce

Mustard ⊘

Proteins

Canned anchovies (in water)

Canned tuna (skipjack and tongol in water recommended for low mercury)

Canned sardines (in water)

Canned wild salmon (in water)

Baking

Almond flour and other nut/seed flours ⊘

Applesauce (unsweetened)

Arrowroot flour (also called arrowroot powder or starch)

Baking soda

Gluten-free baking powder ⊘

Carob powder for AIP

Cassava flour

Flaxseed meal

Shredded unsweetened coconut

Organic maple syrup

Dark chocolate (85% and above with minimal ingredients; there are Paleo brands you can find) ⊘

Coconut flour

Raw honey

Pumpkin puree

Sweet potato puree

Medjool dates

Dried prunes

Dried Herbs and Seasonings

Cinnamon

Cloves

Ginger

Sea salt

Black pepper ⊘

Rosemary

Sage

Thyme

Garlic powder

Onion powder

Coriander ⊘

Cumin ⊘

Basil

Dill

Mint

Oregano

Turmeric

Ginger

Vanilla extract (gluten-free extracts or powders)

Fats and Cooking Oils

Coconut butter (sometimes called "manna")

Canned coconut cream

Canned full-fat coconut milk

Extra-virgin olive oil

Avocado oil

Ghee (or grass-fed butter if tolerated) ⊘

Nut/seed butters such as sunflower seed and tahini ⊘

Lard, schmaltz, tallow

Virgin coconut oil

Nuts/Seeds

Pumpkin seeds (pepitas) ⊘

Raw almonds ⊘

Raw cashews ⊘

Other

Collagen peptides

Kombucha (if tolerated)

Aloe vera juice (whole leaf, unsweetened)

Organic teas (green, black ⊘, white ⊘, red, herbal)

Grass-fed gelatin

Fair-trade organic coffee (if tolerated, or decaf) ⊘

Almond milk (without emulsifiers) ⊘

Sparkling mineral water (if tolerated)

Filtered water

Water or coconut water kefir

Coconut water (no additives or sweeteners)

Paleo & AIP-Friendly Freezer Staples

Proteins

Wild shrimp, deveined and peeled

Wild sea scallops

Wild salmon fillets

Wild fillet of sole or any white flat fish

Ground meat, a variety such as beef, bison, lamb, elk (grass-fed)

Chicken breast, drumsticks, wings, thighs (organic, pasture-raised)

Sausage (usually homemade and frozen using ground meat or a trusted brand; always check ingredients)

Bacon (nitrite-, nitrate-, sugar-free)

Pork chops (pasture-raised)

Burger patties (grass-fed red meat and organic pasture-raised poultry such as turkey)

Chicken or turkey cutlets (organic, pasture-raised)

Chicken liver (organic, pasture-raised)

Vegetables

Artichoke hearts

Carrot

Cauliflower rice

Chopped spinach

Butternut squash

Mixed mushrooms

Pearl onions

Broccoli florets

Cauliflower florets

Beets

Mixed vegetables (Paleo-friendly, without corn or beans)

Green peas

Fruits

Berries

Cherries

Pineapple

Mango

Cranberries

INDEX

A

Acid, promoting strong stomach, 11
Alcohol, 17, 20
Alliums, 16
Almond butter
    Cranberry Orange Flourless Muffins, 163
    No-Churn Blueberry Cardamom Nice Cream, 157
Aloe vera, 21
Aloe vera juice, 31
    Lavender Lemonade with Aloe, 179
    Lemon and Ginger Aloe Vera Tonic, 176
Anchovy fillets, in Avocado Caesar Dressing, 140
Animal fats, 16
Animal protein, 14
Anti-inflammatory whole foods, 31–33
Applesauce, in Cranberry Orange Flourless Muffins, 163
Apples, in Sautéed Cinnamon Apples with Yogurt, 154
Artichokes, Lemon Spatchcock Chicken and, 91
Arugula, in Smoked Salmon Salad with Jammy Eggs, 148
Asparagus, in Tuna Niçoise Salad, 143
Autoimmune Protocol (AIP) diet, 19–21, 49
    meal plans, 198–199
Avocado
    Avocado Crema Dressing, 144
    Mango Chicken Jibaritos (Plantain Sandwiches), 105
    Massaged Kale Caesar, 140

B

Bacon
    Chicken, Bacon, Brussels Sprouts, and Squash Skillet, 84
    Irish Colcannon, 126
Basil leaves
    Pesto Dressing, 148
    Pesto Primavera Veggie Noodles with Shrimp, 115
    Salsa Verde, 192
Béchamel Sauce, Dairy-Free, 108
Beef. See also Ground beef
    "Cheesecake" Stuffed Sweet Potatoes, 98
    Green Goddess Skillet, 87
    Instant Pot Beef Stew, 72
    Rib Eye Steak with Chimichurri, 97
Beets, in Ginger Balsamic Beets and Greens, 134
Bell peppers
    Chicken Pad Thai with Green Papaya Noodles, 147
    Green Coconut Curry Shrimp Soup, 56

Bison
    Greek Stuffed Cabbage Rolls in Lemony Sauce, 112
    Green Goddess Skillet, 87
    Pastelón (Puerto Rican Casserole), 106
    Picadillo with Plantain Rice, 80
Blueberries (frozen), in No-Churn Blueberry Cardamom Nice Cream, 157
Bok choy, in Teriyaki Salmon and Bok Choy, 102
Brain-gut connection, 11–13
Broccoli
    Creamy Chicken and Broccoli Bake, 111
    Shrimp and Broccoli, 103
Broth(s), 31
    Basic broth recipe, 182
    benefits of, 31, 42
    Bone Broth Garlic Kale, 121
    Bone Broth Kale, 121
    Bone Broth Mangú with Salsa Verde, 130
    Bone Broth Ramen, 68
    Bone Broth recipe, 182
    Chicken, Bacon, Brussels Sprouts, and Squash Skillet, 84
    Chicken Marbella, 83
    Creamy Chicken and Mushroom Risotto, 88
    Creamy Ginger, Pear, and Butternut Squash Soup, 64
    Gold Bone Broth Latte, 169
    Green Goddess Skillet, 87
    Green Minestrone Soup with Sausage, 67
    Hot Cocoa Bone Broth, 166
    Instant Pot Beef Stew, 72
    Instant Pot Lamb Shanks, 75
    Instant Pot Pernil (Garlic Pulled Pork), 77
    Instant Pot Shredded Chicken, 74
    Italian Wedding Soup, 63
    making, 40
    Moussaka (Greek Eggplant Casserole), 109
    Mushroom and Cauliflower Rice Soup with Chicken, 71
    Pastelón (Puerto Rican Casserole), 106
    Picadillo with Plantain Rice, 80
    starting to drink, 197
Brussels sprouts, in Chicken, Bacon, Brussels Sprouts, and Squash Skillet, 84
Butternut squash
    Chicken, Bacon, Brussels Sprouts, and Squash Skillet, 84
    Creamy Ginger, Pear, and Butternut Squash Soup, 64

C

Cabbage
    Chicken Pad Thai with Green Papaya Noodles, 147
    Fermented Coleslaw, 184–185
    Greek Stuffed Cabbage Rolls in Lemony Sauce, 112
    Meat Hash with Kale and Cabbage, 94
Capers
    Chicken Marbella, 83
    Chimichurri, 191
    Tuna Niçoise Salad, 143
Cardamom, 31
Cardamom pods
    Rooibos Chai, 177
    Rose-Cardamom Marshmallow Root Tea, 170
Carrots
    Basic Broth, 182
    Bone Broth Ramen, 68
    Chicken Pad Thai with Green Papaya Noodles, 147
    Chicken Zoodle Soup, 60
    Fermented Coleslaw, 184–185
    Instant Pot Beef Stew, 72
    Instant Pot Lamb Shanks, 75
    Italian Wedding Soup, 63
    Lemon Spatchcock Chicken and Artichokes, 91
    Lemony Greek Fisherman's Soup, 59
    Mushroom and Cauliflower Rice Soup with Chicken, 71
    Shrimp and Broccoli, 103
    Slow Cooker Bone Broth, 182
    Sweet-and-Sour Meatballs with Roasted Cauliflower, 101
Cashew butter
    Cranberry Orange Flourless Muffins, 163
    No-Churn Blueberry Cardamom Nice Cream, 157
Casseroles
    Creamy Chicken and Broccoli Bake, 111
    Moussaka (Greek Eggplant Casserole), 109
    Pastelón (Puerto Rican Casserole), 106
    Spaghetti Squash Pastitsio(Greek Baked Ziti), 108
Cauliflower (mashed)
    Creamy Mashed Cauliflower with Mushroom Gravy, 123
    Instant Pot Lamb Shanks, 75
    Pastelón (Puerto Rican Casserole), 106
Cauliflower florets
    "cheese" sauce, 188

Irish Colcannon, 126
Sweet-and-Sour Meatballs with
    Roasted Cauliflower, 101
Cauliflower rice
    Creamy Chicken and Mushroom
        Risotto, 88
    Italian Wedding Soup, 63
    Mushroom and Cauliflower Rice Soup
        with Chicken, 71
    Veggie Confetti Rice, 133
Chai, Rooibos, 177
"Cheese" sauce
    "Cheesecake" Stuffed Sweet
        Potatoes, 98
    Creamy Chicken and Broccoli Bake,
        111
    Dairy-Free Cauliflower Béchamel
        Sauce, 108
    Moussaka (Greek Eggplant
        Casserole), 109
    recipe, 188
    Spaghetti Squash Pastitsio (Greek
        Baked Ziti), 108
Chewing your food, 11, 24, 25
Chicken. See also Ground poultry
    Basic Broth, 182
    Chicken, Bacon, Brussels Sprouts, and
        Squash Skillet, 84
    Chicken Marbella, 83
    Chicken Pad Thai with Green Papaya
        Noodles, 147
    Chicken Zoodle Soup, 60
    Creamy Chicken and Broccoli Bake,
        111
    Crispy Roasted Chicken Thighs with
        Salsa Verde, 100
    Instant Pot Shredded Chicken, 74
    Lemon Spatchcock Chicken and
        Artichokes, 91
    Mango Chicken Jibaritos (Plantain
        Sandwiches), 105
    Massaged Kale Caesar, 140
    Mushroom and Cauliflower Rice Soup
        with Chicken, 71
Chicken bones, in Slow Cooker Bone Broth,
    183. See also Broth(s)
Chicken feet
    Basic Broth, 182
    Slow Cooker Bone Broth, 183
Chicken liver, in Mushroom Truffle Pâté, 194
Chimichurri sauce
    Crispy Baked Sweet Potato Fries with,
        122
    recipe, 191
    Rib Eye Steak with Chimichurri, 97
Chocolate, 20
    Hot Cocoa Bone Broth, 166
    Tahini Caramel Bars, 160

Cilantro
    Avocado Crema Dressing, 144
    Chicken Pad Thai with Green Papaya
        Noodles, 147
    Green Coconut Curry Shrimp Soup, 56
    Mango Chicken Jibaritos (Plantain
        Sandwiches), 105
    Mango Salsa, 193
    Pastelón (Puerto Rican Casserole),
        106
    Picadillo with Plantain Rice, 80
    Salsa Verde, 192
    Tropical Shrimp Salad, 144
Cinnamon, 31
Clean 15 list, 27
Cloves, 31
    Rooibos Chai, 177
Cobbler, Peach, 152
Cocoa powder, Hot Cocoa Bone Broth, 166
Coconut
    Coconut Custard Pie, 158–159
    Strawberry and Cream Yogurt
        Parfaits, 155
Coconut cream
    "cheese" sauce, 188
    Mushroom Truffle Pâté, 194
    No-Churn Blueberry Cardamom Nice
        Cream, 157
Coconut milk
    Coconut Custard Pie, 158–159
    Gold Bone Broth Latte, 169
    Green Coconut Curry Shrimp Soup, 56
    Green Goddess Dressing, 87
    Hot Cocoa Bone Broth, 166
    Instant Pot Coconut Yogurt, 187
    Pumpkin Spice Turmeric Latte, 173
    Rooibos Chai, 177
    Rosemary Parsnip Puree, 137
Coconut oil, 31
Coconut yogurt
    Coconut Custard Pie, 158–159
    Creamy Chicken and Broccoli Bake,
        111
    Green Goddess Skillet, 87
    Peach Cobbler with, 152
    recipe, 187
    Sautéed Cinnamon Apples with
        Yogurt, 154
    Strawberry and Cream Yogurt
        Parfaits, 155
Coffee, 20
Coleslaw, Fermented, 184
Constipation, 197
Cooking tips and tricks, 50
Cooking tools, 53
Cranberries, in Cranberry Orange Flourless
    Muffins, 163

Cruciferous vegetables, 16
Cucumber(s)
    Smoked Salmon Salad with Jammy
        Eggs, 148
    Tropical Shrimp Salad, 144
    Tuna Niçoise Salad, 143
Curcumin. See Turmeric

D

Dairy, 17
Dates, in Tahini Caramel Bars, 160
Dehydration, 46
Diarrhea, 197
Digestion, everyday practices for optimal,
    23–46
Digestive process, 11–13
Dirty Dozen list, 27
Dressings
    Avocado Caesar Dressing, 140
    Avocado Crema Dressing, 144
    Green Goddess Dressing, 87
    Pesto Dressing, 148

E

Egg-Lemon Sauce, Lemony Greek
    Fisherman's Soup, 59
Eggplant, in Moussaka (Greek Eggplant
    Casserole), 109
Eggs, 16, 20. See also Soft-boiled eggs
    Herb-Stuffed Frittata, 95
    sourcing quality, 27
Environmental Working Group (EWG), 29
Enzyme-rich fruits, 32
Epigenetics, 9
Exercise, 38

F

Fasting, 26
Fennel bulb, in Green Minestrone Soup with
    Sausage, 67
Fennel seeds, 32
    Italian Wedding Soup, 63
Fermented Coleslaw
    Massaged Kale Caesar, 140
    recipe, 184
Fermented foods, 17, 32, 42
Fish and seafood
    Crispy Golden Salmon, 92
    Green Coconut Curry Shrimp Soup, 56
    Lemony Greek Fisherman's Soup, 59
    Pesto Primavera Veggie Noodles with
        Shrimp, 115
    Shrimp and Broccoli, 103
    sourcing quality, 27, 29
    Teriyaki Salmon and Bok Choy, 102
    Tropical Shrimp Salad, 144
    Tuna Niçoise Salad, 143

Food(s)
 anti-inflammatory whole, 31–33
 to avoid, 17
 eating a variety of, 35–36
 eating nutrient-dense, 27, 29
 in Paleo diet, 16–17
 preparing for easy digestion, 47
 shopping for, 29–30
Food additives, 20
Food by Mars (blog), 9
Food sensitivities, 20, 35
Frittata, Herb-Stuffed, 95
Frozen foods, 29
Frozen vegetables, in Pesto Primavera
 Veggie Noodles with Shrimp, 115
Fruit(s), 16
 enzyme-rich, 32
 sourcing quality, 27
Fungi, edible, 16

G

Garlic pulled pork. See Instant Pot Pernil
 (Garlic Pulled Pork)
Ginger/ginger juice
 benefits of, 32
 Bone Broth Ramen, 68
 Chicken Pad Thai with Green Papaya
  Noodles, 147
 Creamy Ginger, Pear, and Butternut
  Squash Soup, 64
 Ginger Balsamic Beets and Greens,
  134
 Green Coconut Curry Shrimp Soup, 56
 Lemon and Ginger Aloe Vera Tonic, 176
 Pumpkin Spice Turmeric Latte, 173
 Shrimp and Broccoli, 103
 Shrimp Marinade, 103
 Sweet-and-Sour Meatballs with
  Roasted Cauliflower, 101
 Teriyaki Salmon and Bok Choy, 102
Gluten, 17
Grains, 17
Green beans
 Fasolakia (Haricots Verts in Tomato
  Sauce), 129
 Green Minestrone Soup with Sausage,
  67
 Tuna Niçoise Salad, 143
Green curry paste, in Green Coconut Curry
 Shrimp Soup, 56
Green Goddess Dressing, 87
Grocery shopping, 29–30
Ground beef
 Greek Stuffed Cabbage Rolls in
  Lemony Sauce, 112
 Italian Wedding Soup, 63
 Meat Hash with Kale and Cabbage, 94
 Pastelón (Puerto Rican Casserole),
  106
 Picadillo with Plantain Rice, 80
 Spaghetti Squash Pastitsio (Greek
  Baked Ziti), 108

Ground pork
 Green Minestrone Soup with Sausage,
  67
 Italian Wedding Soup, 63
Ground poultry
 Creamy Chicken and Mushroom
  Risotto, 88
 Green Goddess Skillet, 87
 Green Minestrone Soup with Sausage,
  67
 Meat Hash with Kale and Cabbage, 94
 Sweet-and-Sour Meatballs with
  Roasted Cauliflower, 101
Gut bacteria, 34, 35, 42
Gut-brain connection, 11–13, 21
Gut health and healing, 8–9, 21

H

Healing journey, 8–9
Health practitioner, working with your, 49
Herbs, 16
High-fat fruits, 16
Hydration, 26, 45, 197

I

Icons, meaning of recipe, 50
Instant Pot Beef Stew, 72
Instant Pot Coconut Yogurt, 187
Instant Pot Lamb Shanks, 75
Instant Pot Pernil (Garlic Pulled Pork)
 Bone Broth Ramen, 68
 recipe, 77
Instant Pot Shredded Chicken, 74
Intestinal permeability. See Leaky gut

J

"Junk" foods, 43–44

K

Kale
 Bone Broth Garlic Kale, 121
 Bone Broth Kale, 121
 Bone Broth Ramen, 68
 Green Minestrone Soup with Sausage,
  67
 Herb-Stuffed Frittata, 95
 Irish Colcannon, 126
 Massaged Kale Caesar, 140
 Meat Hash with Kale and Cabbage, 94
 Pesto Primavera Veggie Noodles with
  Shrimp, 115
 Veggie Confetti Rice, 133
Kelp noodles, in Bone Broth Ramen, 68
Kitchen tools, 53

L

Lamb (ground)
 Greek Stuffed Cabbage Rolls in
  Lemony Sauce, 112
 Moussaka (Greek Eggplant
  Casserole), 109
 Spaghetti Squash Pastitsio (Greek
  Baked Ziti), 108

Lamb Shanks, Instant Pot, 75
Lattes
 Gold Bone Broth Latte, 169
 Pumpkin Spice Turmeric Latte, 173
Lavender
 benefits of, 32
 Lavender Lemonade with Aloe, 179
Leafy greens, 16
Leaky gut, 12, 35
Leeks, in Green Minestrone Soup with
 Sausage, 67
Legumes, 17
Lemonade, Lavender, 179
Lemongrass, in Green Coconut Curry
 Shrimp Soup, 56
Lemon juice, 32
Lettuce
 Mango Chicken Jibaritos (Plantain
  Sandwiches), 105
 Tropical Shrimp Salad, 144
 Tuna Niçoise Salad, 143

M

Mango salsa
 Mango Chicken Jibaritos (Plantain
  Sandwiches), 105
 recipe, 193
 Tostones with Mango Salsa (Fried
  Green Plantains), 118
 Tropical Shrimp Salad, 144
Marshmallow root, 21
 about, 32
 Marshmallow Root Tea, Rose-
  Cardamom, 170
Meal plans, 198–199
Meatballs
 Italian Wedding Soup, 63
 Sweet-and-Sour Meatballs with
  Roasted Cauliflower, 101
Meats. See also individual types of meats
 eating quality, 27
 organ, 32
Mercury content, in fish and seafood, 27
Microbiome, 14, 21, 35
Mindful eating, 24–25, 197
Mint leaves
 Nettle Tea Mojito Mocktail, 174
 Pineapple, Lime, and Mint Sorbet, 156
Mixed greens
 Smoked Salmon Salad with Jammy
  Eggs, 148
Muffins, Cranberry Orange Flourless, 163
Mushrooms, 16
 Bone Broth Ramen, 68
 Creamy Chicken and Mushroom
  Risotto, 88
 Creamy Mashed Cauliflower with
  Mushroom Gravy, 123
 Mushroom and Cauliflower Rice Soup
  with Chicken, 71
 Mushroom Truffle Pâté, 194

N

Nettle Tea Mojito Mocktail, 174
Nightshade sensitivity, 20
Nori sheet slices, in Bone Broth Ramen, 68
Nutrient-dense food, sourcing, 27, 29
Nutritional yeast
    "Cheese" sauce, 188
    Creamy Chicken and Mushroom
        Risotto, 88
    Pesto Primavera Veggie Noodles with
        Shrimp, 115
    Smoked Salmon Salad with Jammy
        Eggs, 148
    Spaghetti Squash Pastitsio (Greek
        Baked Ziti), 108
Nuts and seeds
    eliminating, 20, 21
    in the Paleo diet, 17
    soaking, 47

O

Offal/organ meats, 16, 32
Oils
    sourcing quality, 27
    types to avoid/eliminate, 17, 20
    types to cook with, 17
Olives
    Chicken Marbella, 83
    Pastelón (Puerto Rican Casserole),
        106
    Picadillo with Plantain Rice, 80
    Tuna Niçoise Salad, 143
Orange zest, in Cranberry Orange Flourless
    Muffins, 163
Outdoors, spending time, 14

P

Paleo diet
    Autoimmune Protocol Diet, 19–21
    benefits of, 19
    diet template, 19, 20, 21
    explained, 14–17
    meal plans, 198–199
Paleo swaps, 51
Papaya, in Chicken Pad Thai with Green
    Papaya Noodles, 147
Parsley
    Chimichurri, 191
    Fasolakia (Haricots Verts in Tomato
        Sauce), 129
    Greek Stuffed Cabbage Rolls in
        Lemony Sauce, 112
    Instant Pot Lamb Shanks, 75
    Italian Wedding Soup, 63
Parsnips
    Irish Colcannon, 126
    Rosemary Parsnip Puree, 137
Peach Cobbler, 152
Pears, in Creamy Ginger, Pear, and
    Butternut Squash Soup, 64
Peas, in Green Minestrone Soup with
    Sausage, 67

Pepitasan topping
    Creamy Chicken and Broccoli Bake,
        111
    Creamy Chicken and Mushroom
        Risotto, 88
Pesto, kale, 115
Pie, Coconut Custard, 158–159
Pineapple, Lime, and Mint Sorbet, 156
Plantain Rice, Picadillo with, 80
Plantains
    Bone Broth Mangú with Salsa Verde,
        130
    Mango Chicken Jibaritos (Plantain
        Sandwiches), 1005
    Pastelón (Puerto Rican Casserole),
        106
    Picadillo with Plantain Rice, 80
    Tostones with Mango Salsa (Fried
        Green Plantains), 118
Plant foods, 14
Plant oils, 17
Pork. See also Bacon; Ground pork
    Bone Broth Ramen, 68
    Instant Pot Pernil (Garlic Pulled Pork),
        77
Poultry. See also Chicken; Ground poultry
    eating quality, 27
    in Paleo diet, 16
Prebiotics, 14, 34, 42
Probiotics, 14, 17, 42
Processed foods, 17
Prosciutto, in Herb-Stuffed Frittata, 95
Prunes, in Chicken Marbella, 83

R

Radishes
    Massaged Kale Caesar, 140
    Smoked Salmon Salad with Jammy
        Eggs, 148
    Tuna Niçoise Salad, 143
Raisins
    Pastelón (Puerto Rican Casserole),
        106
    Picadillo with Plantain Rice, 80
Ramen, Bone Broth, 68
Red meat, 16. See also Bacon; Beef; Bison;
    Ground pork; Pork
Refined sugar, 17
Root vegetables, 16
Rosebuds, in Rose-Cardamom
    Marshmallow Root Tea, 170
Rutabagas
    Instant Pot Beef Stew, 72
    Lemon Spatchcock Chicken and
        Artichokes, 91
    Lemony Greek Fisherman's Soup, 59
    Pesto Primavera Veggie Noodles with
        Shrimp, 115

S

Salads
    Chicken Pad Thai with Green Papaya
        Noodles, 147

    Massaged Kale Caesar, 140
    Smoked Salmon Salad with Jammy
        Eggs, 148
    Tropical Shrimp Salad, 144
    Tuna Niçoise Salad, 143
Salmon
    Crispy Golden Salmon, 92
    Smoked Salmon Salad with Jammy
        Eggs, 148
    Teriyaki Salmon and Bok Choy, 1002
Salsa, Mango, 193
Salsa verde
    Bone Broth Mangú with Salsa Verde,
        130
    Crispy Baked Sweet Potato Fries with,
        122
    Crispy Roasted Chicken Thighs with
        Salsa Verde, 100
    recipe, 192
    Sauces. See also "Cheese" sauce;
        Chimichurri sauce
    AIP-Friendly Sauce, 147
    Dairy-Free Cauliflower Béchamel
        Sauce, 108
    Egg-Lemon Sauce, 59
    Lemon Cream Sauce, 112
    Sweet-and-Sour Sauce, 101
Seafood and shellfish, 16
Seafoodwatch.org, 29
Sea vegetables, 16
Seeds. See Nuts and seeds
Shirataki noodles, in Bone Broth Ramen, 68
Shrimp
    Green Coconut Curry Shrimp Soup, 56
    Pesto Primavera Veggie Noodles with
        Shrimp, 115
    Shrimp and Broccoli, 103
    Tropical Shrimp Salad, 144
Sleep, 14, 37
Snacks, store-bought ready-made, 51
Snap peas, in Green Coconut Curry Shrimp
    Soup, 56
Soft-boiled eggs
    Bone Broth Ramen, 68
    Massaged Kale Caesar, 140
    Smoked Salmon Salad with Jammy
        Eggs, 148
    Tuna Niçoise Salad, 143
Sorbet, Pineapple, Lime, and Mint, 156
Soups
    Bone Broth Ramen, 68
    Chicken Zoodle Soup, 60
    Creamy Ginger, Pear, and Butternut
        Squash Soup, 64
    Green Coconut Curry Shrimp Soup, 56
    Green Minestrone Soup with Sausage,
        67
    Italian Wedding Soup, 63
    Lemony Greek Fisherman's Soup, 59
    Mushroom and Cauliflower Rice Soup
        with Chicken, 71
Soy, 17
Spaghetti Squash Pastitsio (Greek Baked
    Ziti), 108

Spices, 16, 20
Spinach
Bone Broth Ramen, 68
    Creamy Chicken and Mushroom
       Risotto, 88
    Green Minestrone Soup with Sausage,
       67
    Italian Wedding Soup, 63
    Tuna Niçoise Salad, 143
Star anise, Rooibos Chai, 177
Stews, Instant Pot Beef, 72
Strawberries, in Strawberry and Cream
  Yogurt Parfaits, 155
Stress management, 38–39
Sugar cravings, 44
Sunflower seed butter, in Chicken Pad Thai
  with Green Papaya Noodles, 147
Sweet-and-Sour Sauce, 101
Sweet peppers, in Green Coconut Curry
  Shrimp Soup, 56
Sweet potato(es). *See also* White sweet
  potato(es)
    "Cheesecake" Stuffed Sweet
       Potatoes, 98
    Crispy Baked Sweet Potato Fries, 122
    Green Goddess Skillet, 87
    Veggie Confetti Rice, 133

T

Tahini, in Tahini Caramel Bars, 160
Tea
    Nettle Tea Mojito Mocktail, 174
    Rooibos Chai, 177
    Rose-Cardamom Marshmallow Root
       Tea, 170
Teriyaki Sauce, in Teriyaki Salmon and Bok
  Choy, 102
Tigernut flour
    Peach Cobbler, 152
    Tahini Caramel Bars, 160
Tigernut milk, in Pumpkin Spice Turmeric
  Latte, 173

Tomatoes
    Fasolakia (Haricots Verts in Tomato
       Sauce), 129
    Moussaka (Greek Eggplant
       Casserole), 109
    Tomato paste/puree
    Instant Pot Lamb Shanks, 75
    Moussaka (Greek Eggplant
       Casserole), 109
    Pastelón (Puerto Rican Casserole),
       106
    Picadillo with Plantain Rice, 80
    Spaghetti Squash Pastitsio (Greek
       Baked Ziti), 108
Tuna Niçoise Salad, 143
Turmeric, 34
    Creamy Chicken and Broccoli Bake,
       111
    Creamy Ginger, Pear, and Butternut
       Squash Soup, 64
    Crispy Golden Salmon, 92
    Gold Bone Broth Latte, 169
    Green Coconut Curry Shrimp Soup, 56
    Pumpkin Spice Turmeric Latte, 173
    Shrimp and Broccoli, 103
Turnips
    Instant Pot Beef Stew, 72
    Lemon Spatchcock Chicken and
       Artichokes, 91

V

Vagus nerve, 13, 39
Vegetable oils, 20
Vegetables. *See also* individual types of
  vegetables
    eating a variety of, 36
    preparing for easy digestion, 47–48
    sourcing quality, 27
Veggie confetti rice
    Instant Pot Lamb Shanks, 75
    recipe, 133

W

Water, filtering, 46
Water intake, 45
Water, lemon, 32
Whipped coconut cream
    Coconut Custard Pie, 158–159
    Peach Cobbler with, 152
White sweet potato(es)
    Coconut Custard Pie, 158–159
    Creamy Chicken and Mushroom
       Risotto, 88
    Greek Stuffed Cabbage Rolls in
       Lemony Sauce, 112
    Mushroom and Cauliflower Rice Soup
       with Chicken, 71

Y

Yogurt. *See* Coconut yogurt

Z

Zucchini or zoodles
    Chicken Zoodle Soup, 60
    Green Coconut Curry Shrimp Soup, 56
    Green Minestrone Soup with Sausage,
       67